NAFLD Diet Cookbook

Quick & Simple Fatty Liver-Friendly Recipes for Liver Health, Weight Loss, and Wellness with Healthy Fats, Lean Proteins, and Fiber-Rich Foods.

ANITA JACOB

Copyright © 2024 by Anita Jacob. All rights reserved.

No part of this publication may be reproduced, distributed, or transmitted in any form or by any means, including photocopying, recording, or other electronic or mechanical methods, without the prior written permission of the publisher, except in the case of brief quotations embodied in critical reviews and certain other noncommercial uses permitted by copyright law.

Legal Disclaimer

The content in this book comes from a credible source and is correct based on the author's knowledge, belief, expertise, and information. Before making any substantial dietary changes or beginning on any diet or exercise-related lifestyle program, the reader should contact with their professional healthcare practitioner as needed. The author and publisher of this work accept no responsibility for any negative effects or repercussions stemming from the usage of any of the diets detailed here.

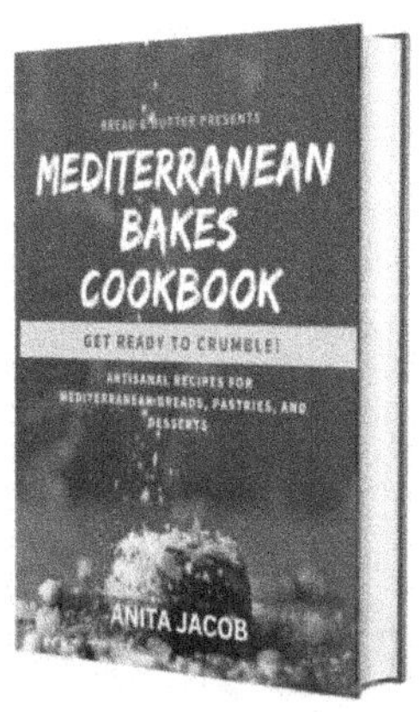

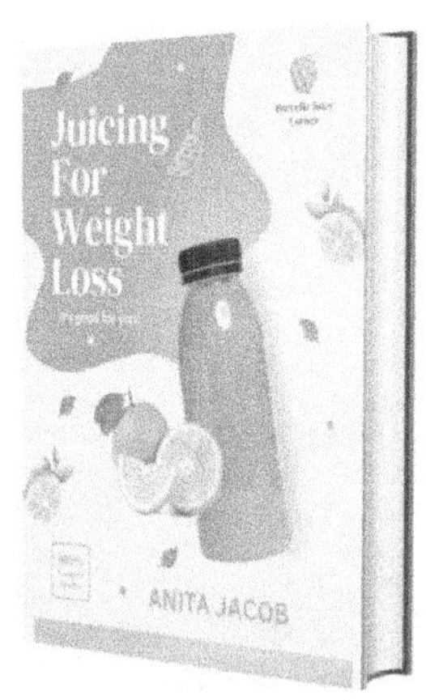

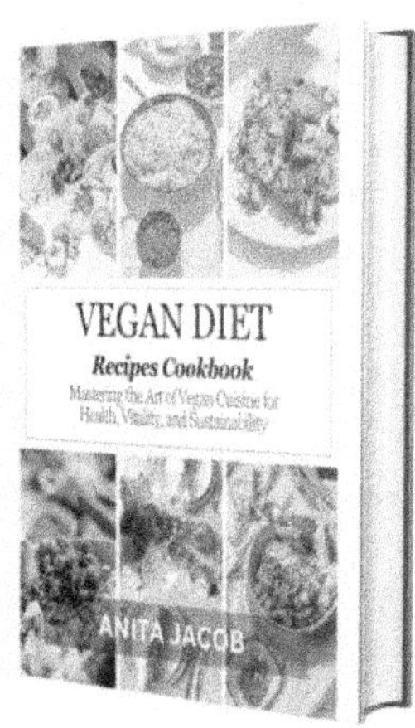

BAKES JUICING VEGAN DIET

TABLE OF CONTENTS

My journey into the field of culinary healing and health is not only a professional venture, but also a very personal one, rooted in the difficulties and successes of the most significant person in my life—my mother, Megan. This tale is more than just the production of a cookbook; it's a journey through sorrow, hope, and the transformational power of nutrition that has led me to become an advocate for the significant influence our food can have on our health.

The narrative begins in the shadow of my mother's health issues, a scary maze with no apparent escape. Megan's illness threw a veil over our family, transforming our days into a whirlwind of doctor appointments, pharmaceutical trials, and an unceasing hunt for solutions. It was a period of uncertainty, but we also discovered a light of hope. A sympathetic doctor advised we take a more holistic approach, focusing on nutrition's ability to not only manage but also enhance Megan's health concerns.

My mother's health gradually improved as we made big modifications to her diet, which was nothing short of a revelation. It was real evidence of food's ability to heal, and it helped solidify my increasing confidence in the power of dietary choices. Megan's path from illness to greater health demonstrated a simple yet deep truth: the food we eat can be an aid in negotiating the difficulties of health and wellbeing.

This understanding spurred me into the depths of the culinary world, where I began to investigate the complex link between food, health, and cooking. My approach was holistic, realizing that a really healthy lifestyle goes beyond simply choosing the proper components; it is about how we interact with food, from preparation to consumption. This attitude formed the foundation of my work, guiding me as I strove to provide realistic, effective guidance to anyone wishing to improve their health via eating.

As my education and experience grew, so did my desire to reach out and inspire a larger audience. The worldwide upheaval caused by the COVID-19 epidemic underlined the significance of providing accessible, practical advice on healthy living. During this period of seclusion and introspection, I decided to embrace the power of the written word, beginning on a quest to develop cookbooks that contained more than simply recipes. My books were created as comprehensive guides to a better living, combining personal tales, nutritional insights, and a wealth of practical advice to make healthy eating a fun and important part of daily life.

The recipes I've written are a monument to my path, which was distinguished by resilience, strong optimism, and a firm confidence in food's restorative power. From seeing my mother Megan's change to being a beacon of hope for others, my journey has been a clear example of how educated food choices can have a huge impact on our health and happiness.

In my job as a nutritionist, I want to be more than simply a source of nutritional guidance; I want to be a companion on the journey to wellness, providing empathy, support, and a celebration of each step toward a healthy life. My aim is clear: to enable people to take responsibility of their health, one meal at a time, and discover the joy and freedom that comes with living a fulfilling life.

The legacy I hope to leave behind is measured not by the recipes I've made or the advice I've offered, but by the lives I've touched and impacted by my devotion. My transformation from a spectator to my mother's recovery journey to a coach for others confirms my conviction in the healing power of food. Nutrition, in my opinion, goes beyond science; it becomes an art form, an expression of love, and a path to a more happy, healthier life.

Through " NAFLD Diet Cookbook: Quick & Simple Recipes for Liver Health, Weight Loss, and Wellness with Healthy Fats, Lean Proteins, and Fiber-Rich Foods.," I welcome you to join me at a table full of healing and hope. This is more than just a cookbook; it invites you to embark on a wellness journey and discover the transformational power of thoughtful, educated eating. Let's go on a delightful, nutritious journey to health and vitality, showing that the finest medicine is there on our plates.

By Dr. Ruth Ford, Leading Hepatologist and a Friend of Mine.

Non-Alcoholic Fatty Liver Disease (NAFLD) is a substantial health concern that impacts a considerable proportion of the world's population. An acquaintance and eminent hepatologist, Dr. Ruth Ford, frequently discusses the profound effect that diet has on liver health. NAFLD comprises a variety of liver conditions from simple fat accumulation to more severe forms like Non-Alcoholic Steatohepatitis (NASH), which can progress to cirrhosis and liver cancer. The function of diet in the management and potentially reversal of this disease is crucial.

The foundation of combating NAFLD lies in dietary management, emphasizing the reduction of calories from lipids and sugars. In addition to reducing caloric intake, it is vital to select foods that offer nutritional advantages. It is crucial to consume a diet abundant in fruits, vegetables, whole carbohydrates, and lean proteins. Antioxidants and fiber, which are abundant in these foods, aid in the reduction of hepatic fat and the improvement of insulin sensitivity.

Moreover, selecting the proper lipids is crucial. Unsaturated fats, such as those found in salmon, nuts, and olive oils, should be prioritized as they help to reduce inflammation and enhance lipid profiles. On the other hand, saturated and trans fats—commonly found in processed and fried foods—should be minimized due to their potential to increase hepatic obesity.

Sugar intake, particularly fructose from processed foods and saccharine beverages, must be carefully managed. High fructose levels are linked to increased liver lipids, inflammation, and a heightened risk of developing more severe liver diseases.

Additionally, micronutrients are vital to liver health. Vitamin E, for instance, has shown potential in enhancing liver function in people with NASH, and many individuals with NAFLD have a deficiency in vitamin D. Considering supplementation might be beneficial but should be done under professional guidance.

Hydration is another basic yet crucial aspect of a liver-friendly diet. Water assists in metabolizing and eliminating impurities from the liver, supporting overall metabolic processes.

The recipes included in this cookbook are designed by Anita Jacob, a nutritionist, with the aim of making meal preparation both straightforward and beneficial for liver health. Each recipe integrates liver-friendly ingredients and is accompanied by comprehensive nutritional information, empowering readers to make informed dietary choices.

These dietary adjustments, while focused on liver health, also enhance overall wellness. They assist in managing weight, reducing the risk of type 2 diabetes, enhancing heart health, and boosting metabolic functions.

In addition to dietary modifications, regular physical activity and effective weight management are vital in managing NAFLD. These lifestyle adjustments complement each other, increasing liver function and ensuring long-term health benefits.

Through this cookbook, the objective is to not only offer delectable recipes but also to provide education and motivation for making healthful lifestyle choices. By integrating these meals into daily routines, readers are taking proactive measures towards improved liver health and enhanced overall wellness. With a commitment to these principles, each recipe becomes more than just a meal; it is a part of a vital voyage towards health and longevity.

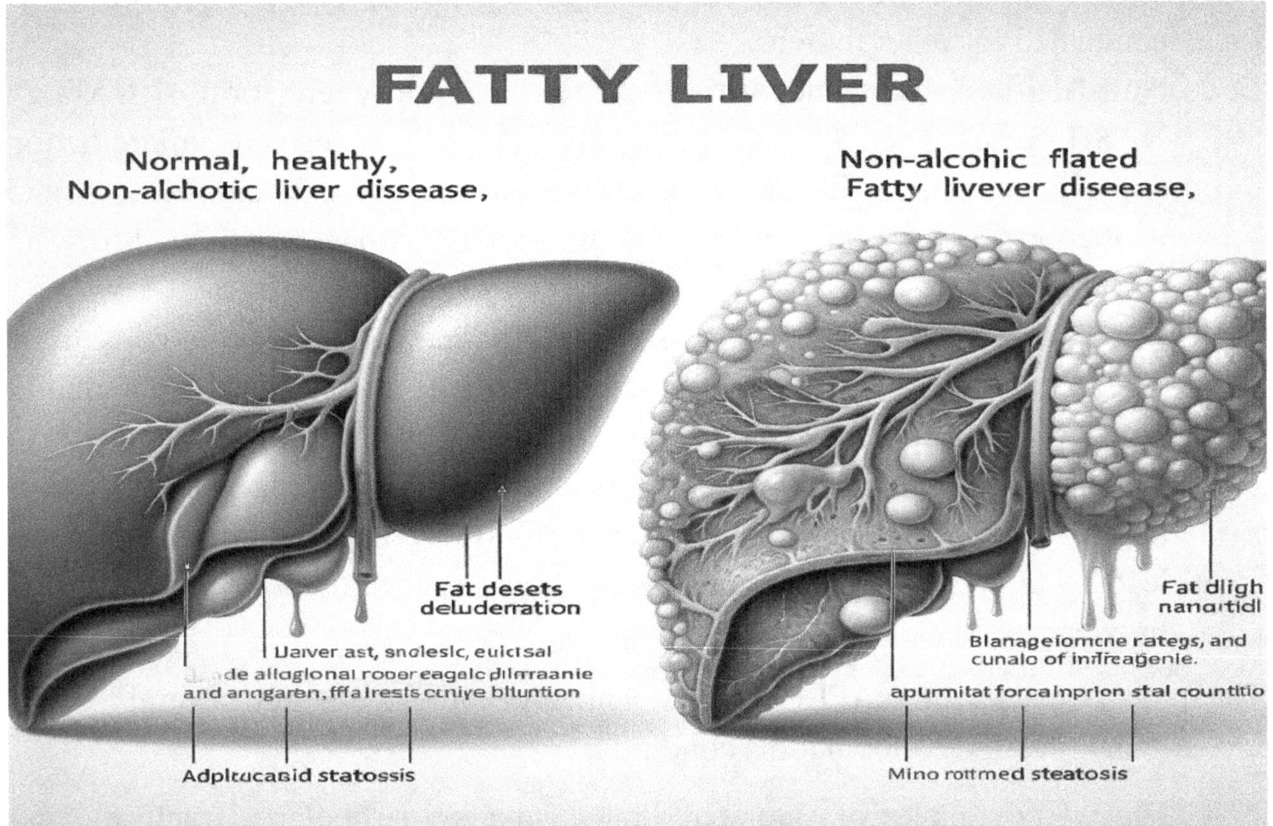

What is Non-Alcoholic Fatty Liver Disease?

Non-Alcoholic Fatty Liver Disease (NAFLD) is the most prevalent liver disorder in the world today, afflicting approximately 25% of the global population. It represents a variety of liver conditions that do not result from alcohol consumption but rather from excess fat deposited in liver cells. This fat accumulation can cause inflammation and injury, potentially leading to more serious liver diseases, such as Non-Alcoholic Steatohepatitis (NASH), cirrhosis, and even liver cancer.

NAFLD is predominantly associated with metabolic syndromes such as obesity, type 2 diabetes, and hyperlipidemia. It often develops in individuals who are overweight or obese, but it can also affect people with normal weight who have excess abdominal fat or other metabolic risk factors.

The Disease Typically Progresses Through Several Stages:

1. **Simple Fatty Liver (Steatosis):** At this initial stage, fat accumulates in the liver cells. This stage is usually innocuous and often reversible with lifestyle

changes. Most individuals with uncomplicated fatty liver do not experience any symptoms and the condition might only be discovered during tests conducted for other reasons.

2. **Non-Alcoholic Steatohepatitis (NASH):** A more severe form of NAFLD, NASH occurs when the fat accumulation in the liver leads to inflammation and liver cell injury. This stage can progress to more severe complications and is often associated with fibrosis, where excessive connective tissue forms up in the liver.
3. **Fibrosis:** During fibrosis, the persistent inflammation in the liver leads to the formation of scar tissue. This stage can still be managed and potentially reversed with appropriate dietary and lifestyle changes.
4. **Cirrhosis:** This advanced stage occurs when scar tissue replaces healthy liver tissue and impairs liver function. Cirrhosis is severe and often irreversible, leading to various health complications and a substantially increased risk of liver cancer.

The precise causes of NAFLD are not entirely understood, but several factors increase the risk of developing this condition:

- **Diet:** High intake of saturated lipids, sugars (particularly fructose), and refined carbohydrates.
- **Obesity:** Particularly the presence of excessive abdominal fat.
- **Insulin Resistance:** Where the body's cells do not respond effectively to insulin.
- **High Blood Sugar:** Indicative of prediabetes or type 2 diabetes.
- **High Levels of Lipids in The Blood:** Particularly high levels of triglycerides.

Detecting NAFLD often involves a combination of blood tests, imaging investigations, and sometimes liver biopsies. Liver function tests can indicate abnormalities, but imaging studies like ultrasound, CT scans, or MRIs are more effective in showing obesity in the liver. In uncertain cases, a liver biopsy may be conducted to corroborate the diagnosis and assess the severity of liver damage.

Management of NAFLD Focuses Largely on Lifestyle Adjustments. Key Interventions Include:

- **Dietary Adjustments:** Reducing calorie intake and adopting a diet abundant in vegetables, fruits, whole cereals, and lean proteins. It is crucial to minimize the intake of saturated fats, trans fats, and refined carbohydrates.
- **Weight Loss:** Losing 5-10% of body weight can substantially reduce liver lipids and inflammation.
- **Exercise:** Regular physical activity helps eliminate triglycerides and reduce liver obesity.
- **Control Of Diabetes and Cholesterol:** Managing these conditions can help mitigate the progression of NAFLD.

Preventing NAFLD involves maintaining a healthy weight, remaining active, and consuming a balanced diet. Regular check-ups with a healthcare provider can also help detect and manage risk factors early.

The Importance of Diet in Managing NAFLD

Diet plays a pivotal role in the management of Non-Alcoholic Fatty Liver Disease (NAFLD). Given that NAFLD and its more severe form, Non-Alcoholic Steatohepatitis (NASH), are predominantly metabolic conditions, interventions focused on dietary and lifestyle adjustments are crucial for prevention and management. Understanding how certain foods and dietary patterns affect liver health can help in constructing a diet that supports liver function and reduces the risk of disease progression.

Dietary Impact on Liver Health

The liver processes everything we consume and drink and filters out hazardous substances from the blood. An optimal diet helps the liver to function efficiently, whereas a poor diet can lead to fat accumulation, inflammation, and liver injury. In NAFLD, excess liver fat is associated with insulin resistance, obesity, and aberrant lipid profiles, which diet directly influences.

Key Dietary Principles for Managing NAFLD

1. **Reduce Caloric Intake:** For those with NAFLD, managing caloric intake is essential to reduce liver obesity. Many studies suggest that even a modest weight loss (about 5-10% of body weight) can help reduce liver fat, enhance inflammation, and decrease the risk of fibrosis.

2. **Focus on Healthy Fats:** Replacing saturated and trans lipids with monounsaturated and polyunsaturated fats can enhance liver health. Foods's rich in omega-3 fatty acids, such as fish, almonds, and seeds, are particularly beneficial as they help reduce hepatic fat levels and inflammation.

3. **Increase Fiber Intake:** High-fiber foods such as fruits, vegetables, whole cereals, and legumes not only help maintain a healthy weight but also enhance insulin sensitivity. Fiber assists in digestion and can help to delay the absorption of sugar, keeping blood glucose levels stable.

4. **Limit Sugars and Refined Carbohydrates:** Diets high in sugars, particularly fructose, and refined carbohydrates can exacerbate hepatic fat accumulation. Avoiding sugary drinks, sweets, and white bread can help prevent increases in blood sugar and reduce the burden on the liver.

5. **Moderate Protein Intake:** Adequate protein intake is vital for liver repair and preventing muscle loss. Lean sources of protein like poultry, fish, tofu, and legumes are recommended over red meat, which can be high in saturated fat.

Practical Tips for Implementing Dietary Changes

- **Plan Meals Ahead:** Meal planning is a beneficial method to control portions and ensure a balanced intake of nutrients. Preparing home-cooked dishes allows for greater control over ingredients and portion sizes.

- **Read Food Labels:** Being informed about the nutritional content of foods can aid in making healthier choices. Look for foods low in saturated fats and sugars while high in fiber and healthful lipids.

- **Stay Hydrated:** Water plays a crucial role in assisting the liver to filter out toxins. Keeping hydrated helps maintain liver health and assists in metabolism.

- **Regular Monitoring:** Regular check-ups with a healthcare provider can help monitor the effects of dietary changes on liver health and overall metabolism.

Impact of Dietary Changes on Overall Health

While the dietary adjustments mentioned are targeted at enhancing liver health, they also offer extensive benefits for overall health. These modifications can help manage weight, reduce the risk of type 2 diabetes, lower cholesterol levels, and enhance cardiovascular health.

Moreover, implementing these dietary principles can lead to enhanced energy levels, better sleep, and a general sense of well-being. The holistic benefits of a balanced diet extend beyond liver health, influencing every aspect of life.

Support Throughout Your Journey

For those commencing on this path, note that changes in diet and lifestyle might take time to show results. Patience and consistency are essential. It is also beneficial to seek support from dietitians, nutritionists, and medical professionals who can provide guidance tailored to individual health requirements.

In this cookbook, you will find a compilation of recipes that adhere to these dietary principles, offering delectable, easy-to-prepare dishes designed to support liver health and overall wellness. Each recipe is crafted to provide optimum nutritional benefit, enabling you to manage NAFLD effectively while enjoying your meals.

Latest Research and Developments (as of 2024)

Non-Alcoholic Fatty Liver Disease (NAFLD) remains a subject of significant medical research and interest due to its increasing prevalence and potential to progress to more severe liver diseases. In recent years, research efforts have intensified, leading to new insights into its pathogenesis, diagnosis, and treatment. Here, we provide a summary of the most notable advancements and developments in the field as of 2024, intending to give readers a clear view of the current landscape and future directions in NAFLD management.

Advances in Understanding Genetic Influences

Recent investigations have deepened our comprehension of the genetic factors contributing to NAFLD. Researchers have identified specific genetic markers that may predict susceptibility to the disease, particularly variants in genes that influence lipid metabolism, insulin resistance, and fibrosis development. These genetic insights are crucial as they could lead to more personalized approaches in treating and managing NAFLD based on individual genetic profiles.

Improved Diagnostic Techniques

Diagnosing NAFLD has traditionally relied on liver biopsies, an invasive procedure. However, the latest advancements include non-invasive imaging technologies and biomarkers that can accurately diagnose and assess the severity of liver injury without the need for a biopsy. Enhanced imaging techniques such as FibroScan, which measures liver stiffness, and MRI-based proton density fat fraction (MRI-PDFF) assessments provide detailed insights into the quantity of fat and fibrosis in the liver. Additionally, novel blood tests that can detect specific biomarkers associated with liver injury and fibrosis are under development, promising simpler, speedier, and safer diagnostic options.

Dietary Interventions and Nutritional Insights

Nutritional research continues to play a crucial role in managing NAFLD. Studies in 2024 have highlighted the impact of specific dietary components more explicitly. For instance, the influence of polyunsaturated fatty acids (PUFAs) and their positive effects on liver health have been underlined. Diets abundant in omega-3 fatty acids are shown to substantially reduce liver fat and inflammation in NAFLD patients.

Another area of interest is the gut-liver axis and its implications for NAFLD. Researchers are investigating how alterations in gastrointestinal microbiota can impact liver health. Probiotics, prebiotics, and a fiber-rich diet have been noted to enhance intestinal flora, which in turn helps reduce liver fat and inflammation.

Pharmacological Developments

While lifestyle modifications remain the cornerstone of NAFLD management, pharmacological treatments have also seen impressive advancements. Several new drugs are in various phases of clinical trials, targeting distinct aspects of NAFLD pathophysiology such as insulin resistance, lipid metabolism, and liver fibrosis. Drugs like GLP-1 agonists, which were initially used for diabetes management, have shown promise in reducing liver obesity and improving liver function tests in NAFLD patients.

Lifestyle Modifications and Behavioral Health

Understanding the role of behavioral factors in managing NAFLD has acquired traction. Research indicates that sustained lifestyle modifications, including dietary habits, physical activity, and weight management, are essential for the effective treatment of NAFLD. Programs focused on behavioral changes that incorporate regular counseling, peer support groups, and tailored exercise regimens have demonstrated success in improving outcomes for NAFLD patients.

Future Directions

Looking forward, the focus of NAFLD research is transitioning towards a more holistic approach that includes not only treatment but also prevention. Public health initiatives aimed at reducing obesity and diabetes prevalence are anticipated to play a vital role in decreasing the incidence of NAFLD. Furthermore, ongoing studies into the incorporation of artificial intelligence in diagnosing and managing NAFLD promise to revolutionize the field.

With these developments, our comprehension of NAFLD continues to progress, leading to more effective and targeted interventions. As we maintain track of these advancements, it is essential to implement this knowledge to daily practices. This cookbook integrates the latest dietary recommendations and health insights, providing recipes that are not only delectable but also beneficial for liver health and overall well-being. Each recipe here correlates with current research, ensuring that readers have access to the most effective dietary strategies for managing NAFLD. Through informed dietary choices, individuals can substantially influence the fate of their liver health, paving the way for a healthier future

To get access to our exclusive bonuses, simply scan the QR Code below! Enjoy your culinary journey! 😊

THANK YOU FOR YOUR PATRONAGE!!

Fiber plays a pivotal role in digestive health, which is closely linked to liver health. High-fiber diets help regulate blood sugar levels and reduce cholesterol, both of which are advantageous for NAFLD patients.

- **Whole Grains:** Foods like quinoa, barley, and brown rice are excellent sources of fiber and are also abundant in B vitamins, which are essential for metabolism and energy production.
- **Vegetables:** Leafy greens such as spinach, kale, and broccoli are high in fiber and rich in a variety of vitamins and minerals that support liver health and detoxification.
- **Fruits:** While fruits are beneficial, those with NAFLD should choose fruits with a lower fructose content, such as berries, apples, and pears, which provide fiber and antioxidants without excessive sugar.
- **Legumes:** Beans and lentils are not only high in protein and fiber but also contain a range of nutrients that support liver health.

Incorporating These Foods into Your Diet

A balanced diet that includes a variety of nutrients from these categories can significantly impact the management of NAFLD. Regularly incorporating healthy lipids, lean proteins, and fiber-rich foods into your meals can help minimize liver fat, reduce inflammation, and enhance liver function. Each recipe in this cookbook has been meticulously designed to include these essential nutrients, making it simpler for you to prepare delectable, healthy meals that support liver health.

Foods to Avoid: Reducing Risk through Smart Choices

Managing Non-Alcoholic Fatty Liver Disease (NAFLD) involves not just adding beneficial foods to your diet, but also identifying and avoiding those that can exacerbate liver conditions. Understanding which foods to limit or exclude is crucial in regulating the progression of NAFLD and enhancing overall liver health. Here, we emphasize on the categories of foods that should be minimized or avoided to maintain a healthy liver.

Saturated and Trans Fats

High intake of saturated fats and trans fats can contribute to an increase in liver fat, which is a significant factor in the development of NAFLD. These lipids also contribute to cardiovascular disease by elevating harmful LDL cholesterol levels and diminishing beneficial HDL cholesterol.

- **Processed Meats:** Foods like sausages, bacon, and salami are high in saturated lipids and should be ingested sparingly.
- **Fast Food:** Common fast-food items, including burgers, fries, and fried chicken, are often abundant in both saturated and trans fats.
- **Baked Goods:** Commercially produced pastries, biscuits, and cakes typically contain trans fats, which are used to extend shelf life and enhance flavor.

Refined Carbohydrates

Foods high in refined carbohydrates can contribute to increases in blood sugar and insulin levels, which are linked to increased liver fat and inflammation in individuals with NAFLD.

- **White Bread and Pasta:** These are made from refined flour, which has most of its fiber and nutrients removed.
- **Sugary Cereals:** Often laden with added sugars and very little nutritional value, these should be avoided.
- **Snack Foods:** Chips, crackers, and other packaged munchies are usually made with refined flour and may contain trans fats.

Sugars and Sweeteners

High consumption of sugar, particularly fructose, is significantly linked to the development of liver obesity. Foods elevated in added carbohydrates can exacerbate liver inflammation and contribute to weight gain.

- **Sugary Drinks:** Soft drinks, fruit beverages, and energy drinks are significant sources of fructose and should be avoided.
- **Candy and Sweets:** These are dense in sugar and offer little nutritional benefit, directly contributing to hepatic fat accumulation.
- **Sweetened Dairy Products:** Flavored yogurts and ice cream can also be rich in added sugars.

Alcohol

While NAFLD is not caused by alcohol, imbibing can exacerbate liver impairment and interfere with liver function. It is generally advisable for individuals with liver issues to avoid alcohol or consume it only in minimal amounts.

Beer, Wine, and Spirits: All alcoholic beverages can contribute to liver obesity and should be consumed with caution or avoided altogether.

Sodium-Rich Foods

Excessive sodium intake is not directly linked to NAFLD but can contribute to water retention and hypertension, which are risk factors for cardiovascular disease.

- **Canned Soups and Vegetables:** These often contain excessive levels of sodium as a preservative.
- **Salted Snacks:** Chips and pretzels are typically high in sodium.
- **Processed Cheeses and Meats:** These can also contain significant quantities of sodium and should be limited.

Making Smart Dietary Choices

Avoiding these foods requires consistent attention to diet and making informed choices when purchasing and dining out. Reading labels and selecting whole, unprocessed foods can significantly enhance your diet's quality and support your liver health.

By adhering to these dietary guidelines and choosing foods judiciously, you can significantly reduce the risk factors associated with NAFLD. The recipes supplied in the cookbook are designed to align with these principles, allowing you to experience delicious, healthy meals without compromising your liver health.

Regular physical activity and maintaining a healthy weight are also crucial in supporting these dietary efforts, enhancing both liver health and overall well-being.

Reading Food Labels for Better Choices

Understanding how to read food labels is crucial for making healthier dietary choices, particularly for individuals managing conditions like Non-Alcoholic Fatty Liver Disease (NAFLD). A well-informed consumer can better avoid the excess lipids, sugars, and other constituents that contribute to liver issues. Here, we provide a comprehensive guide on how to interpret the information contained on food labels to help you select the best options for a liver-friendly diet.

Start with the Serving Size

Food labels are designed to be informative, detailing the nutrients for a specific serving size. It's crucial to examine the serving size at the top of the label to comprehend how many servings are in each container. This helps to accurately assess the amount of calories and nutrients you will be consuming if you consume one serving or the whole package.

Calories Count

Calories are a measure of how much energy food provides. For those managing NAFLD, monitoring calorie intake is essential, particularly if weight loss is recommended. Compare the calories per serving among similar products and choose the option that corresponds with your dietary requirements without being excessively high.

Understand Macronutrients

The next section on most food labels lists the macronutrients: lipids, carbohydrates, and proteins. For NAFLD, particular attention should be paid to the categories of lipids and carbohydrates.

- **Fats:** Look for items low in saturated lipids and trans fats. Prefer products with higher unsaturated lipids like monounsaturated and polyunsaturated fats. Remember, labels must identify the amounts of each form of fat, helping you avoid those detrimental to liver health.
- **Carbohydrates:** Pay heed to carbohydrates and fiber. High fiber content is advantageous as it assists in digestion and can help control blood sugar levels. Try to select foods with minimal sugar content, notably avoiding those with added carbohydrates.
- **Proteins:** Adequate protein intake is essential for health. Choose foods that provide a decent source of protein which will help with satiety and muscle maintenance.

Look for Sodium and Cholesterol

Both sodium and cholesterol can impact overall health, particularly cardiovascular health. Since NAFLD is associated with increased risk of cardiovascular diseases, selecting foods with lower sodium and cholesterol content is prudent.

Check for Added Sugars

One of the most critical aspects for those with NAFLD is to avoid added carbohydrates. High intake of fructose, in particular, is associated with increased hepatic obesity. Many products now list added carbohydrates on the label, allowing you to see precisely how much sugar has been added to the product beyond what is naturally occurring in the ingredients.

Inspect Ingredient Lists

The ingredients list on a food label is where you can find out what precisely is in your food. Ingredients are enumerated in order of quantity, from highest to lowest. Look for whole foods as the first ingredients and be wary of lengthy lists containing unrecognizable items as this often indicates a high degree of processing.

Nutritional Claims Labels often contain claims like "low-fat," "reduced sodium," or "high fiber." These can help make fast decisions but should not supplant your assessment of the nutrition facts label. Always verify the label to ensure these claims meet your specific dietary requirements.

Special Labels: Organic, Non-GMO, etc.

If your dietary strategy incorporates organic or non-GMO foods, labels are crucial. These certifications can usually be found on the packaging and signify that the food satisfies certain standards regarding its production and processing.

Utilizing Food Labels in Meal Planning

With practice, reading product labels becomes a fast and automatic part of shopping. Use this skill to evaluate products and choose those that best suit into your NAFLD-friendly diet. Planning meals around foods that align with these label-reading strategies can help you maintain a healthy liver and overall body.

By educating yourself on the specifics of food labels, you can exercise significant control over your diet and health. Regularly selecting the correct foods based on accurate label information is a potent tool in managing NAFLD. Each recipe in our cookbook considers these guidelines, ensuring that you can create meals that are not only delectable but also beneficial for your health.

To get access to our exclusive bonuses, simply scan the QR Code below! Enjoy your culinary journey! 😊

THANK YOU FOR YOUR PATRONAGE!!

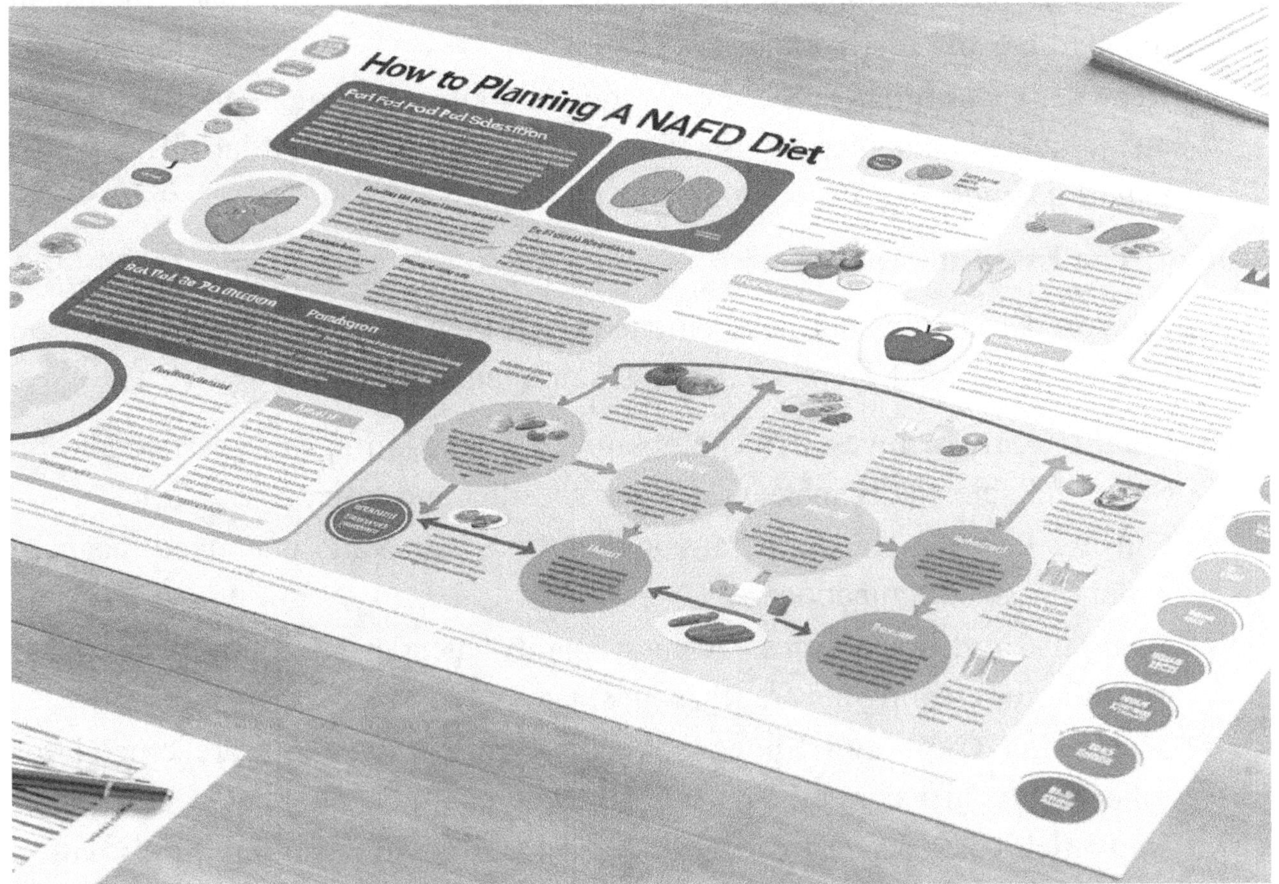

Setting Up Your Kitchen for Success

Creating a kitchen environment that supports your Non-Alcoholic Fatty Liver Disease (NAFLD) diet is vital for assuring day-to-day ease and long-term adherence to a healthy eating plan. A well-organized and adequately supplied kitchen can make the process of preparing nutritious meals both enjoyable and efficient. Here are practical tips for setting up your kitchen to nurture success on your voyage toward liver health.

Organize Your Space

An orderly and well-organized kitchen saves time and reduces tension during meal preparation. Here are a few organizational strategies:

- **Clear the Clutter:** Remove any items you don't use regularly. This includes outdated seasonings, expired foods, and unnecessary kitchen devices.

- **Define Work Zones:** Set up specific areas for preparing, cooking, and cleaning to streamline your culinary process. This approach helps in maintaining an orderly kitchen.
- **Use Clear Containers:** Store dry products like rice, quinoa, and legumes in clear, labeled containers. This setup not only keeps your larder tidy but also makes it simple to see what you have on hand.

Stock Up on Essential Tools

Having the proper instruments can facilitate the cooking process and encourage you to prepare meals at home. Here's a list of essential culinary tools:

- **Quality Knives:** Invest in a chef's knife, a paring knife, and a serrated knife. Sharp, reliable blades make prep work speedier and safer.
- **Cutting Boards:** Have separate boards for produce and uncooked meats to avoid cross-contamination.
- **Blenders and Processors:** A high-quality blender or food processor is essential for creating beverages, soups, and purees.
- **Measuring Cups and Spoons:** Accurate measuring tools are crucial for following recipes correctly, particularly when commencing a new diet.
- **Non-Stick Cookware:** Reduce the need for excessive cooking lipids with a set of non-stick cookware.

Choose Healthy Cooking Methods

The method you cook your food can affect its nutritional content. Emphasize culinary methods that retain nutrients and limit unhealthy fats:

- **Steaming and Boiling:** Excellent for vegetables, these methods do not require lipids and preserve the natural nutrients.
- **Grilling and Broiling:** These techniques allow fat to trickle away from the food and generate a rich, smoky flavor.
- **Sautéing:** Use a small quantity of healthy oil or broth in a non-stick pan for fast and healthy cooking.

Stock Healthful Ingredients

Keeping healthful ingredients on board is key to adhering to a NAFLD-friendly diet. Here are some staples to maintain in your larder, refrigerator, and freezer:

- **Whole Grains:** Brown rice, whole wheat pasta, and quinoa are versatile and rich in fiber.
- **Lean Proteins:** Stock up on fish, poultry, legumes, and tofu to ensure you have plenty of low-fat protein options.
- **Healthy Fats:** Olive oil, avocados, and almonds are excellent sources of healthy fats.
- **Fruits and Vegetables:** Keep a variety of fresh and frozen vegetables and fruits, concentrating on those high in fiber and low in sugar.
- **Spices and Herbs:** Flavor foods with a range of spices and fresh herbs instead of salt.

Create a Supportive Environment

The overall environment in your kitchen should inspire healthful eating:

- **Visibility:** Place fruits and vegetables where you can see them, such as on a countertop dish, to encourage nibbling on healthful options.
- **Accessibility:** Arrange your kitchen so that healthful foods are simple to access, while less healthy options are out of immediate sight.
- **Inspiration:** Decorate your kitchen with items that motivate you, such as cookbooks, culinary guides, or a board with dietary advice and recipes.

By setting up your kitchen for success, you take an important step in supporting your dietary changes for NAFLD management. An organized, well-equipped, and properly supplied kitchen not only simplifies cooking but also helps in maintaining the motivation to adhere to a healthful diet.

Essential Ingredients for a Liver-Friendly Kitchen

Creating dishes that support liver health begins with stocking your kitchen with the appropriate ingredients. A liver-friendly kitchen is armed with nutrients that help reduce inflammation, lower lipid accumulation, and support overall liver function. Here, we guide you through essential ingredients to keep on hand, ensuring every meal contributes to your health and well-being.

Beneficial Fats

- **Fat:** is a crucial element of the diet, even when managing conditions like Non-Alcoholic Fatty Liver Disease (NAFLD). The key is to focus on lipids that support liver health.
- **Olive Oil:** A staple for cookery and dressings, olive oil is abundant in monounsaturated fats, which are advantageous for liver health.
- **Avocados:** These are not only a source of healthful lipids but also fiber and antioxidants.
- **Nuts and Seeds:** Walnuts, almonds, and flaxseeds provide omega-3 fatty acids and fiber, which can help reduce liver inflammation and enhance lipid profiles.

Lean Proteins

Protein is essential for repairing tissues and maintaining a functional immune system. For liver health, it's crucial to choose proteins that are minimal in fat.

- **Fish:** Options like salmon, sardines, and trout are high in omega-3 fatty acids, which are known for their anti-inflammatory properties.
- **Chicken and Turkey:** Opt for skinless poultry to minimize cholesterol intake.
- **Legumes:** Beans, lentils, and legumes are superb plant-based proteins that are also high in fiber.

Whole Grains

Carbohydrates are necessary for vitality, but the type of carbohydrates you choose is crucial. Whole grains are abundant in fiber, which can help manage blood sugar levels and assist in digestion.

- **Brown Rice:** A versatile grain that is a healthier alternative to white rice.
- **Quinoa:** High in protein and all nine essential amino acids, making it an excellent option for plant-based regimens.
- **Oats:** Perfect for breakfast, oats have beta-glucan, a form of fiber that aids in managing cholesterol levels.

Fiber-Rich Fruits and Vegetables

Fruits and vegetables are essential for their vitamins, minerals, and fiber composition, which support overall liver health.

- **Leafy Greens:** Spinach, kale, and swiss chard are high in antioxidants and low in calories.
- **Berries:** Blueberries, strawberries, and raspberries are abundant in antioxidants and can help combat inflammation.
- **Cruciferous Vegetables:** Broccoli, cauliflower, and Brussels sprouts help enhance the liver's natural detoxification enzymes.

Herbs and Spices

Herbs and spices not only add flavor without the extra calories, but many also have health benefits, including support for liver health.

- **Turmeric:** Contains curcumin, known for its anti-inflammatory and antioxidant properties.
- **Garlic:** Helps activate enzymes in the liver which help flush out impurities.
- **Cinnamon:** Can help control blood sugar and decrease the quantity of fat stored in the liver.

Beverages

What you imbibe is just as essential as what you eat when it comes to liver health.

- **Green Tea:** High in antioxidants, green tea can help reduce fat storage in the liver and enhance liver function.
- **Coffee:** If you appreciate coffee, the good news is that moderate coffee consumption has been linked to a lower risk of liver disease.

Condiments and Extras

Opt for condiments that enhance flavor without adding unnecessary sugars or unhealthy lipids.

- **Vinegars:** Such as apple cider and balsamic, can lend character to dishes without many calories.
- **Mustard and Tahini:** These are excellent for condiments and sauces instead of mayonnaise or cream-based products.
- **Low-Sodium Soy Sauce:** A healthier alternative to conventional soy sauce, which can be high in sodium.

Tips for Stocking Your Liver-Friendly Kitchen

- **Prioritize Freshness:** Whenever feasible, choose raw ingredients over processed foods.
- **Read Labels:** Always read food labels to avoid ingredients that are detrimental to liver health such as high fructose corn syrup and added carbohydrates.
- **Plan Your Meals:** Planning helps ensure that you use these ingredients effectively, reducing waste and ensuring that you enjoy a variety of nutrients.

With these essential ingredients, your kitchen will be well-equipped to create meals that are not only delectable but also beneficial for your liver and overall health. Remember, the proper foods can act as medication, assisting to heal and protect your liver against disease.

Weekly Meal Planning and Prep

Effective administration of Non-Alcoholic Fatty Liver Disease (NAFLD) involves not only knowing what to consume but also planning your meals in advance. Weekly meal preparation and prep is a strategy that helps ensure you maintain a balanced diet throughout the week, which is crucial for enhancing liver health and overall wellness. Here we discuss the benefits of meal planning and provide practical advice on how to make meal prep a regular part of your life.

Benefits of Meal Planning

Meal planning has several advantages, notably for individuals managing dietary requirements due to health conditions like NAFLD:

- **Consistency in Healthy Eating:** By planning your meals, you avoid the pitfall of making unwise food choices when you're famished and unprepared.
- **Control Over Ingredients:** Preparing meals yourself enables you to control what goes into your food, ensuring you remain within your dietary guidelines.
- **Time and Cost Efficiency:** Shopping with a list reduces time at the store and minimizes impulsive buys, saving money in the long run.
- **Reduced Stress:** Knowing what you're going to consume in advance can decrease daily decision fatigue and make mealtime enjoyable rather than a chore.

Steps for Successful Meal Planning

- **Assess Your Weekly Schedule:** Look at your week ahead to determine how many dishes you need to prepare. Consider your work schedule, social excursions, and family commitments.
- **Choose Your Recipes:** Select recipes that suit your dietary requirements and that you find enjoyable. It's useful to have a variety of recipes that require various preparation times: some that can be made swiftly and others that might take longer but are worth the effort.
- **Make a Shopping List:** Based on the recipes you've chosen, compile a purchasing list. Organize your list by categories (produce, protein, dairy, etc.) to streamline your purchasing experience.
- **Set Aside Time for Prep:** Dedicate a few hours one or two days a week for meal prep. This might entail chopping vegetables, marinating proteins, or preparing a large quantity of cereals.
- **Store Meals Properly:** Use hermetic containers to store your prepared meals or ingredients. Label the containers with the contents and date to keep track of what you have and ensure it's used before it expires.

Tips for Efficient Meal Prep

- **Batch Cooking:** Cook vast quantities of versatile ingredients. Grains like brown rice or quinoa and proteins like chicken can be cooked in large quantities and used in various recipes throughout the week.
- **Pre-cut Vegetables:** Wash and trim vegetables ahead of time. Store them in clear containers in your refrigerator to make them simple to reach and use.
- **Smart Storage:** Invest in high quality storage containers that can go from the fridge or freezer to the microwave or oven. Glass containers are optimal as they don't retain aromas or stains and are generally safer for reheating food than plastic.
- **Theme Evenings:** Consider theme evenings to facilitate decision-making. For example, Meatless Monday, Taco Tuesday, or Fish Friday. This can add an enjoyable element to meal planning and help streamline the process.

Creating a Flexible Plan

While it's essential to have a plan, it's equally important to remain flexible. Sometimes plans change, and you may not be in the mood for what you've prepared, or you might have remnants that need to be used. Adjust your plan as required while still attempting to meet your nutritional objectives.

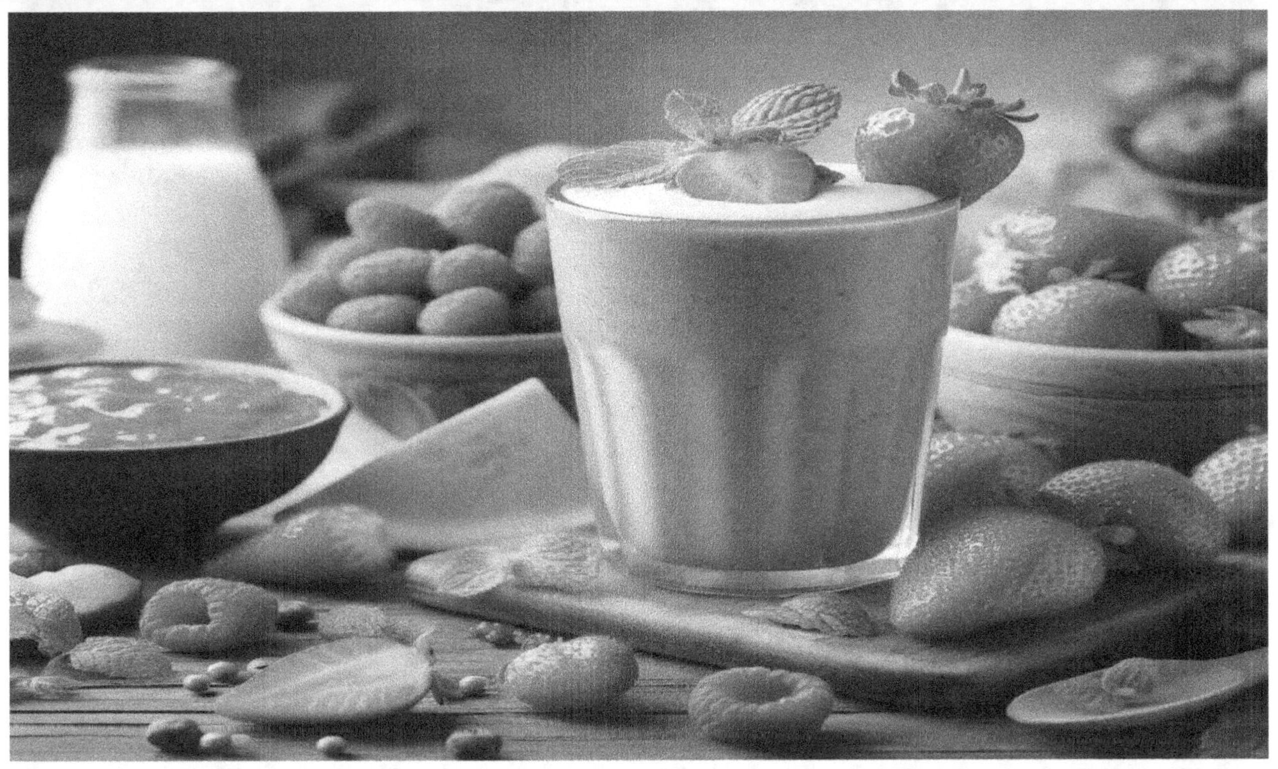

Green Detox Smoothie

Nutritional Information: 250 calories, 5 g protein, 35 g carbohydrates, 10 g fat, 8 g fiber, 15 mg sodium.

Ingredients:

- 1 cup fresh spinach
- 1 small green apple, cored and sliced
- 1/2 avocado
- 1/2 cup cucumber slices
- 1 tablespoon chia seeds
- 1 cup coconut water

Prep Time: 5 minutes, Servings: 1

Instructions:

1. Combine all ingredients in a blender.
2. Blend on high until smooth.
3. Serve immediately.

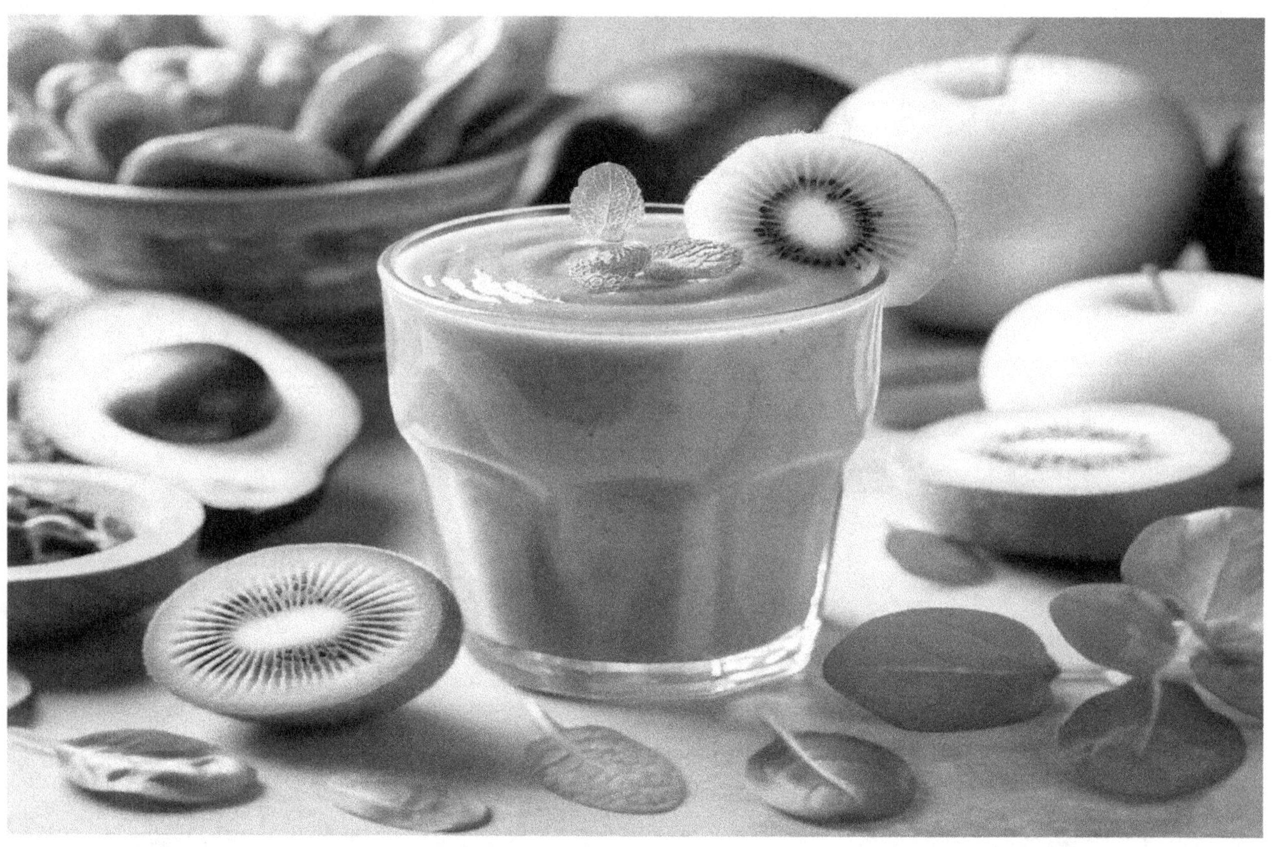

Berry Antioxidant Smoothie

Nutritional Information: 210 calories, 8 g protein, 30 g carbohydrates, 4 g fat, 6 g fiber, 55 mg sodium.

Ingredients:

- 1/2 cup fresh strawberries
- 1/2 cup raspberries
- 1/2 banana
- 1/2 cup Greek yogurt
- 1 teaspoon honey (optional)
- 1/2 cup almond milk

Prep Time: 5 minutes, **Servings**: 1

Instructions:

1. Place all ingredients into a blender.
2. Blend until smooth.
3. Pour into a glass and serve immediately.

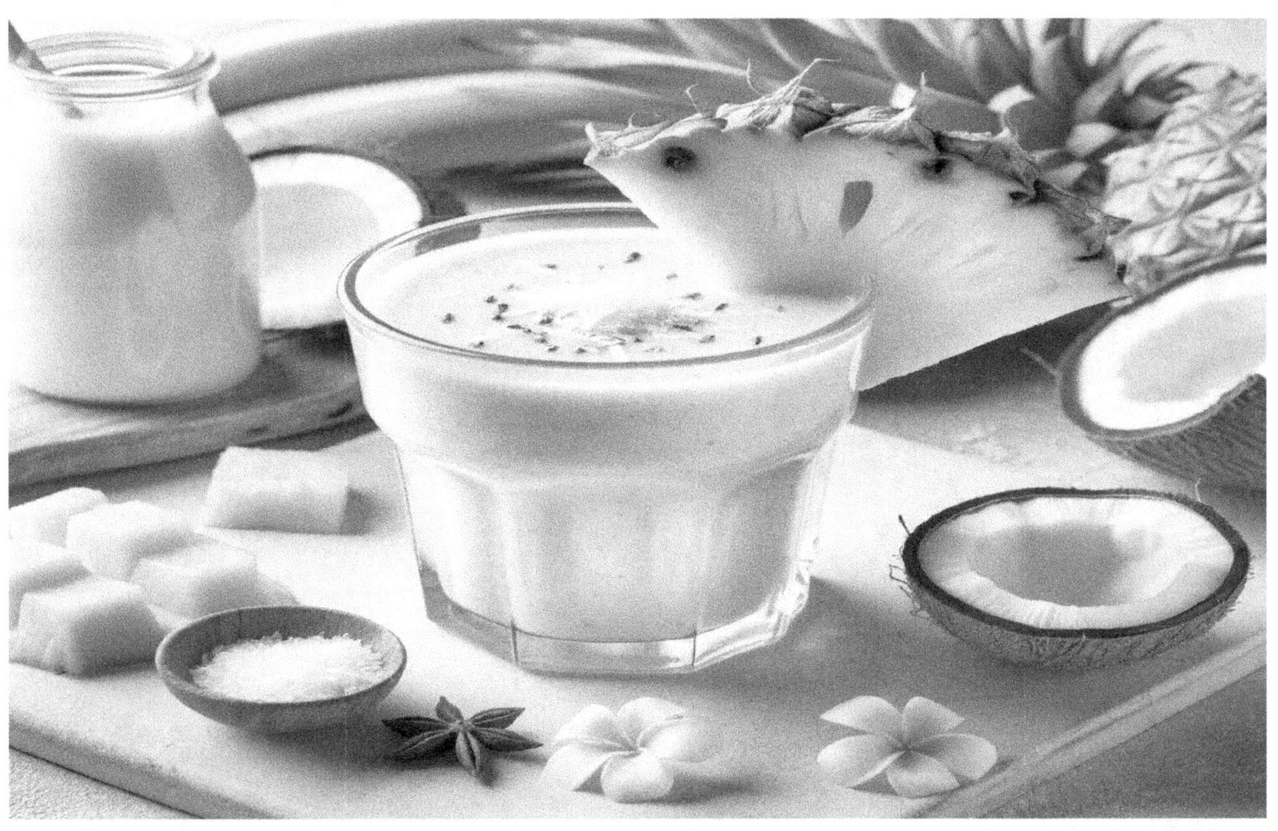

Tropical Digestive Aid Smoothie

Nutritional Information: 180 calories, 2 g protein, 28 g carbohydrates, 7 g fat, 3 g fiber, 30 mg sodium.

Ingredients:

- 1/2 cup pineapple chunks
- 1/2 banana
- 1/4 cup coconut milk
- 1 teaspoon lime juice
- 1/2 teaspoon fresh grated ginger

Prep Time: 5 minutes, **Servings**: 1

Instructions:

1. Add all ingredients to a blender.
2. Blend on high until creamy and smooth.
3. Serve chilled.

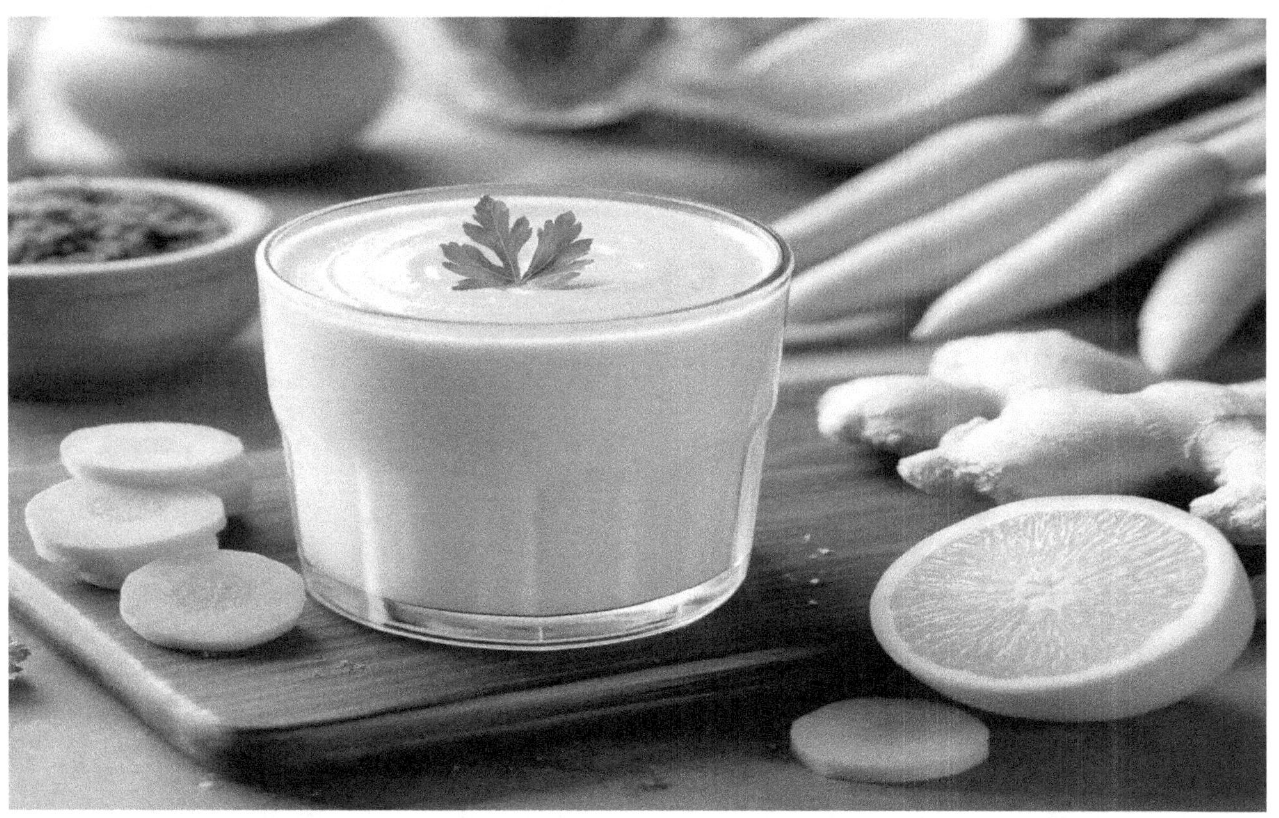

Carrot Ginger Detox Juice

Nutritional Information: 160 calories, 4 g protein, 38 g carbohydrates, 0.5 g fat, 9 g fiber, 70 mg sodium.

Ingredients:

- 4 large carrots, peeled
- 1/2-inch piece of ginger, peeled
- 1 orange, peeled and deseeded
- 1/2 lemon, juice only

Prep Time: 10 minutes, **Servings**: 1

Instructions:

1. Juice all ingredients in a juicer.
2. Stir to combine and pour into a glass.
3. Serve immediately for best nutritional benefits.

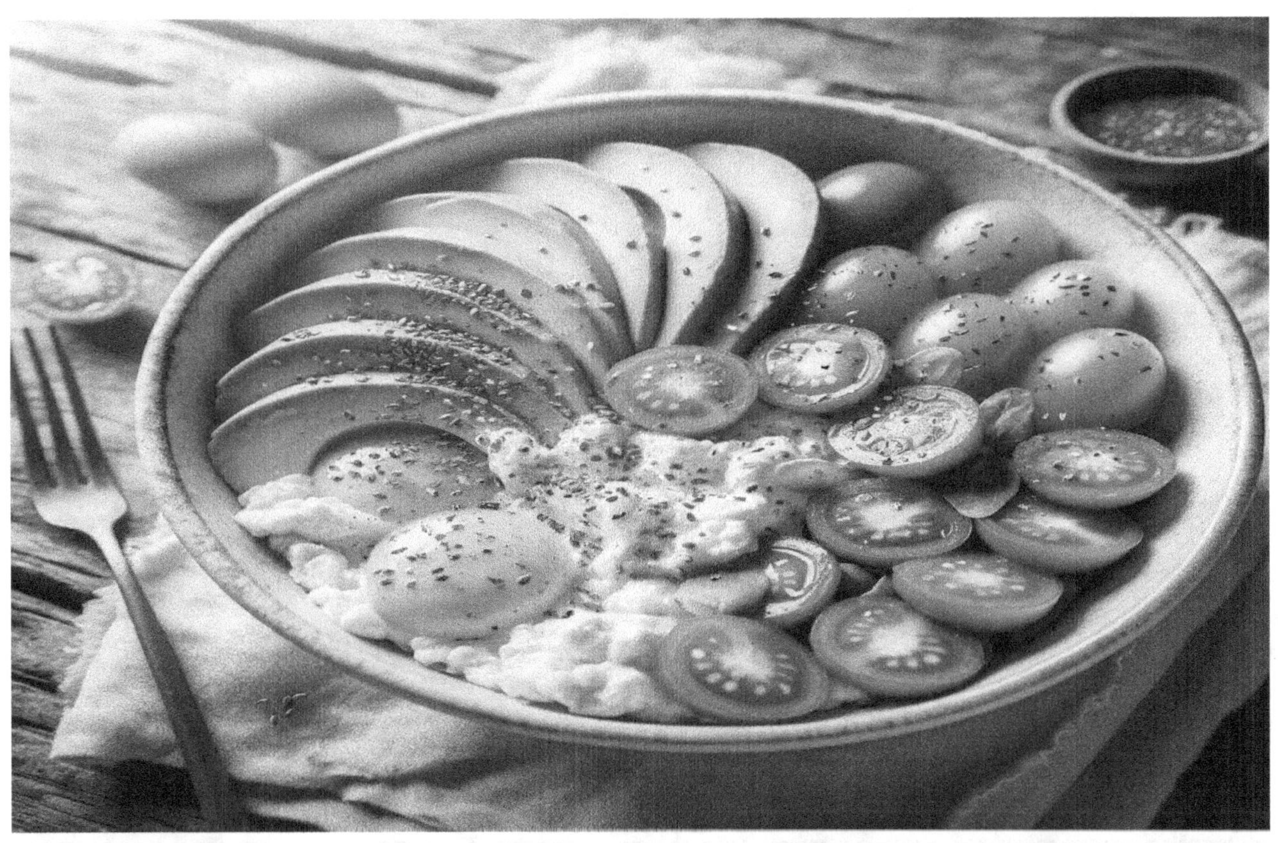

High-Protein Breakfast Bowl

Nutritional Information: Calories: 400, Protein: 20g, Carbohydrates: 18g, Fat: 29g, Fiber: 7g, Sodium: 320mg.

Ingredients:

- 2 large eggs, scrambled
- 1/2 avocado, sliced
- 1/2 cup cherry tomatoes, halved
- 1 tablespoon chia seeds

Prep Time: 5 minutes, **Cook Time**: 5 minutes, **Servings**: 1

Instructions:

1. Cook scrambled eggs to your liking.

2. Arrange the eggs, avocado slices, and cherry tomatoes in a bowl.

3. Sprinkle chia seeds over the top and serve.

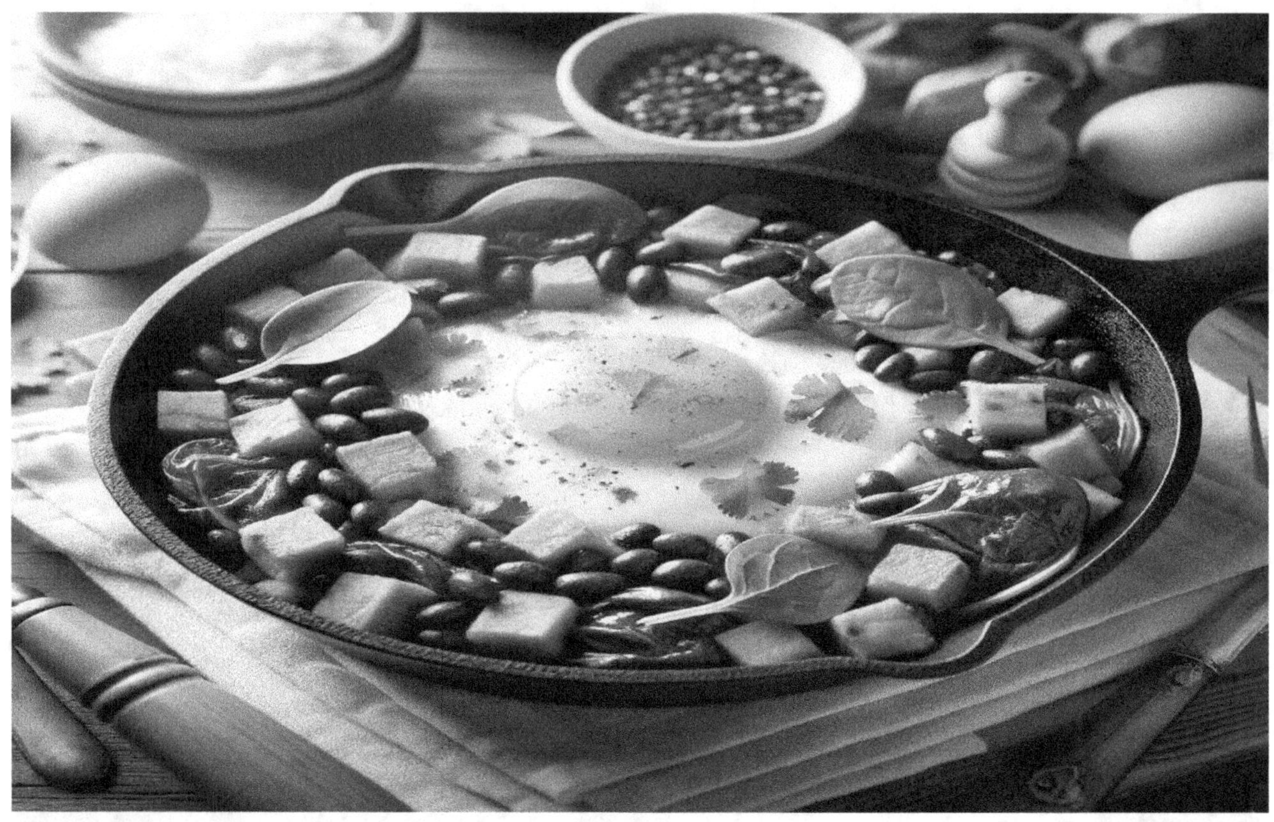

Sweet Potato and Spinach Breakfast Skillet

Nutritional Information: Calories: 350, Protein: 15g, Carbohydrates: 45g, Fat: 14g, Fiber: 10g, Sodium: 400mg.

Ingredients:

- 1 small sweet potato, diced
- 1/2 cup black beans, rinsed and drained
- 1 cup fresh spinach
- 1 large egg
- 1 tablespoon olive oil
- Fresh cilantro for garnish

Prep Time: 10 minutes, **Cook Time**: 15 minutes, **Servings**: 1

Instructions:

1. Heat olive oil in a skillet over medium heat and sauté sweet potatoes until tender.

2. Add black beans and spinach, cooking until spinach is wilted.

3. Make a well in the center and crack the egg into the skillet. Cover and cook until the egg is set.

4. Garnish with cilantro and serve hot.

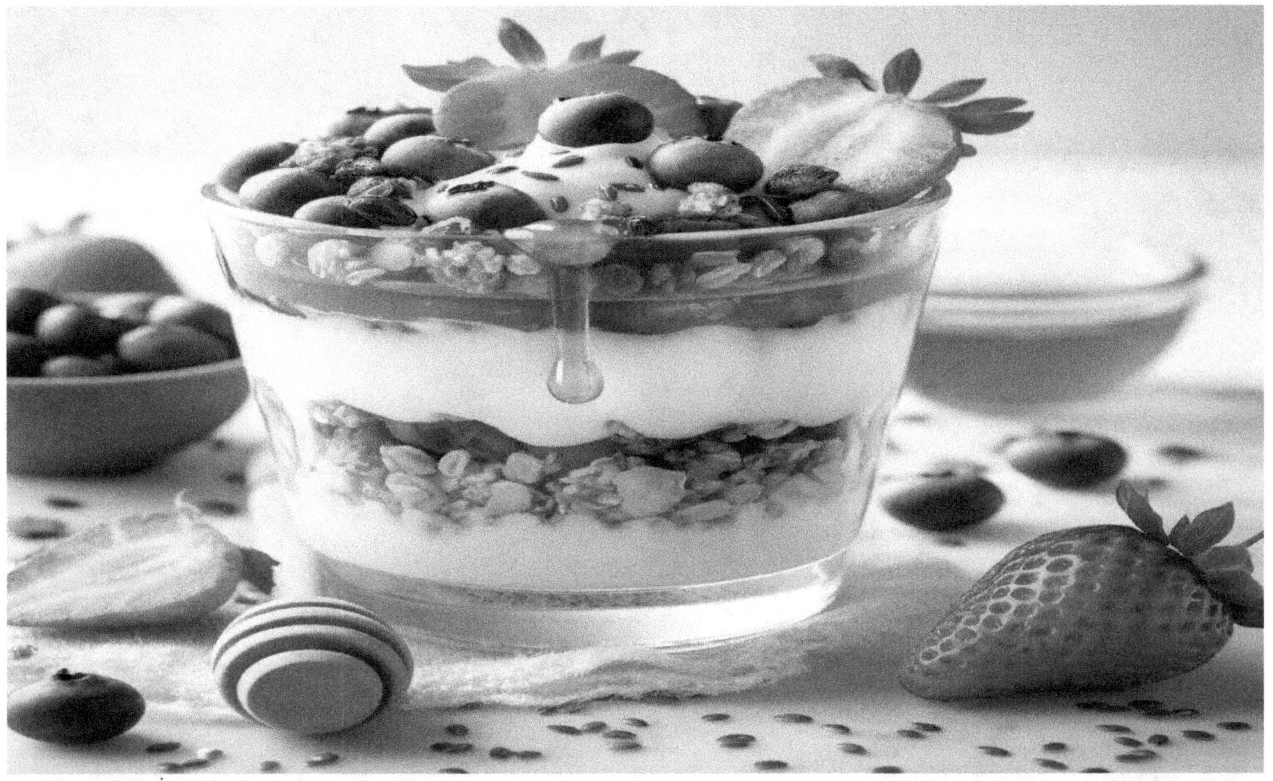

Greek Yogurt Parfait

Nutritional Information: Calories: 280, Protein: 20g, Carbohydrates: 36g, Fat: 8g, Fiber: 5g, Sodium: 85mg.

Ingredients:

- 1 cup Greek yogurt, low-fat
- 1/4 cup granola
- 1/4 cup blueberries
- 1/4 cup sliced strawberries
- 1 teaspoon honey
- 1 tablespoon flax seeds

Prep Time: 5 minutes, **Blend Time**: 0 minutes, **Servings**: 1

Instructions:

1. In a tall glass, layer half of the yogurt, followed by half of the granola, berries, and a drizzle of honey.

2. Repeat the layers with the remaining ingredients.

3. Top with flax seeds and serve immediately.

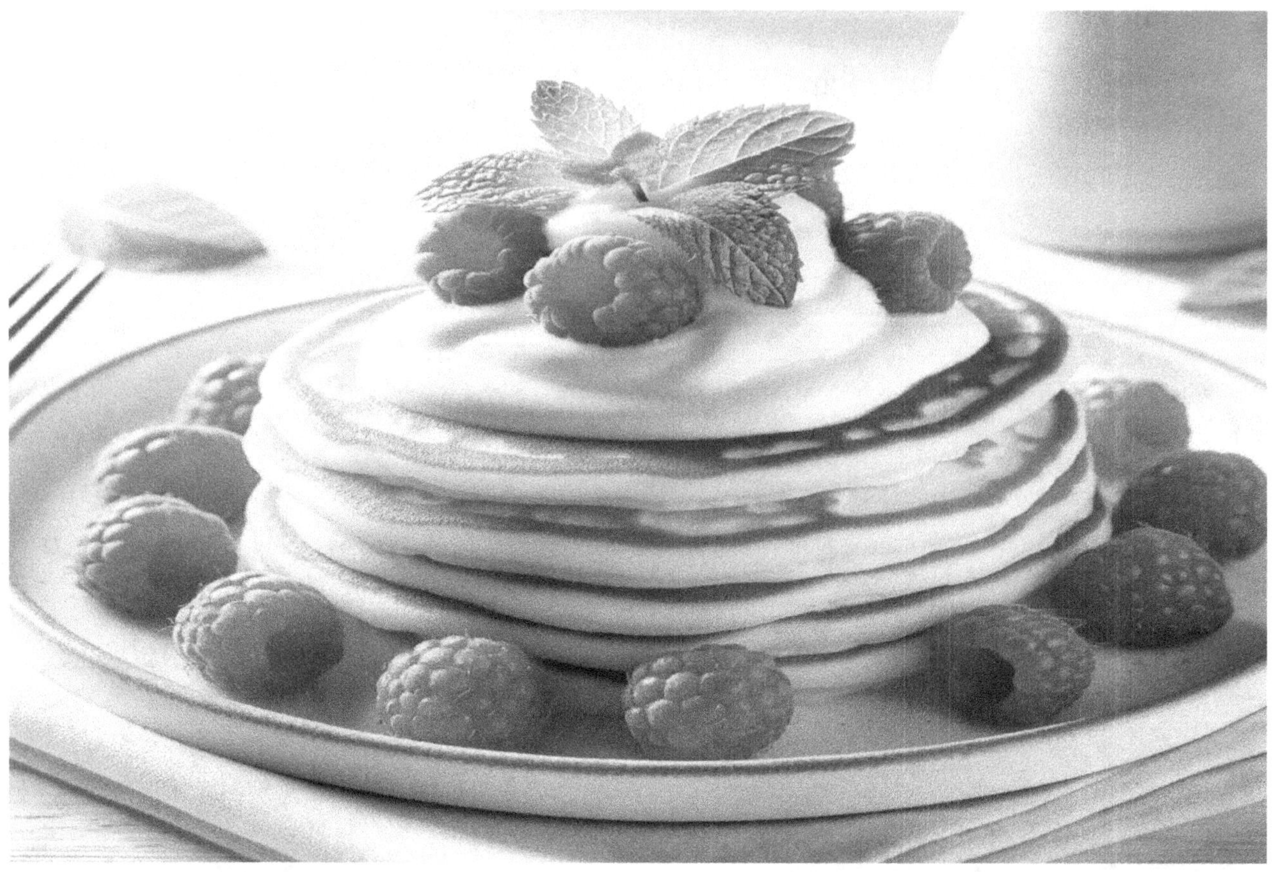

Cottage Cheese Pancakes

Nutritional Information: Calories: 320, Protein: 28g, Carbohydrates: 24g, Fat: 12g, Fiber: 4g, Sodium: 460mg.

Ingredients:

- 1/2 cup cottage cheese
- 1/4 cup whole wheat flour
- 1 egg
- 1 tablespoon low-fat sour cream
- 1/4 cup fresh raspberries
- Mint leaves for garnish

Prep Time: 10 minutes, **Cook Time**: 10 minutes, **Servings**: 1

Instructions:

1. Blend cottage cheese, flour, and egg until smooth.

2. Heat a non-stick skillet over medium heat and pour batter to form small pancakes.

3. Cook until bubbles form on the surface, then flip and cook until golden.

4. Serve with a dollop of sour cream, raspberries, and mint.

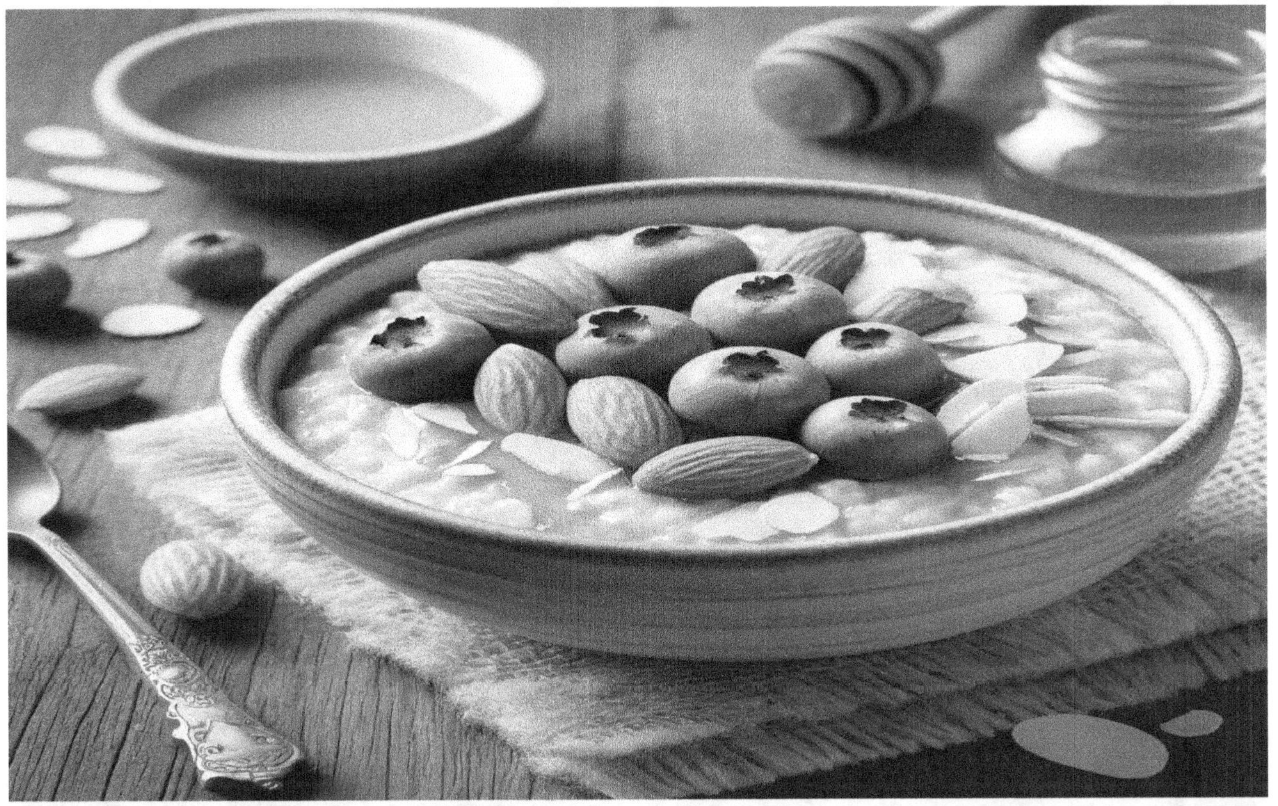

Blueberry Almond Oatmeal

Nutritional Information: 295 calories, 8g protein, 45g carbohydrates, 9g fat, 6g fiber, 30mg sodium.

Ingredients:

- 1/2 cup rolled oats
- 1 cup almond milk
- 1/4 cup blueberries
- 2 tablespoons sliced almonds
- 1 tablespoon honey

Prep Time: 5 minutes, **Cook Time**: 5 minutes, **Servings**: 1

Instructions:

1. In a small pot, bring the almond milk to a boil.

2. Add the rolled oats and reduce heat to a simmer, cook for 5 minutes, stirring occasionally.

3. Remove from heat and stir in blueberries and sliced almonds.

4. Drizzle with honey and serve warm.

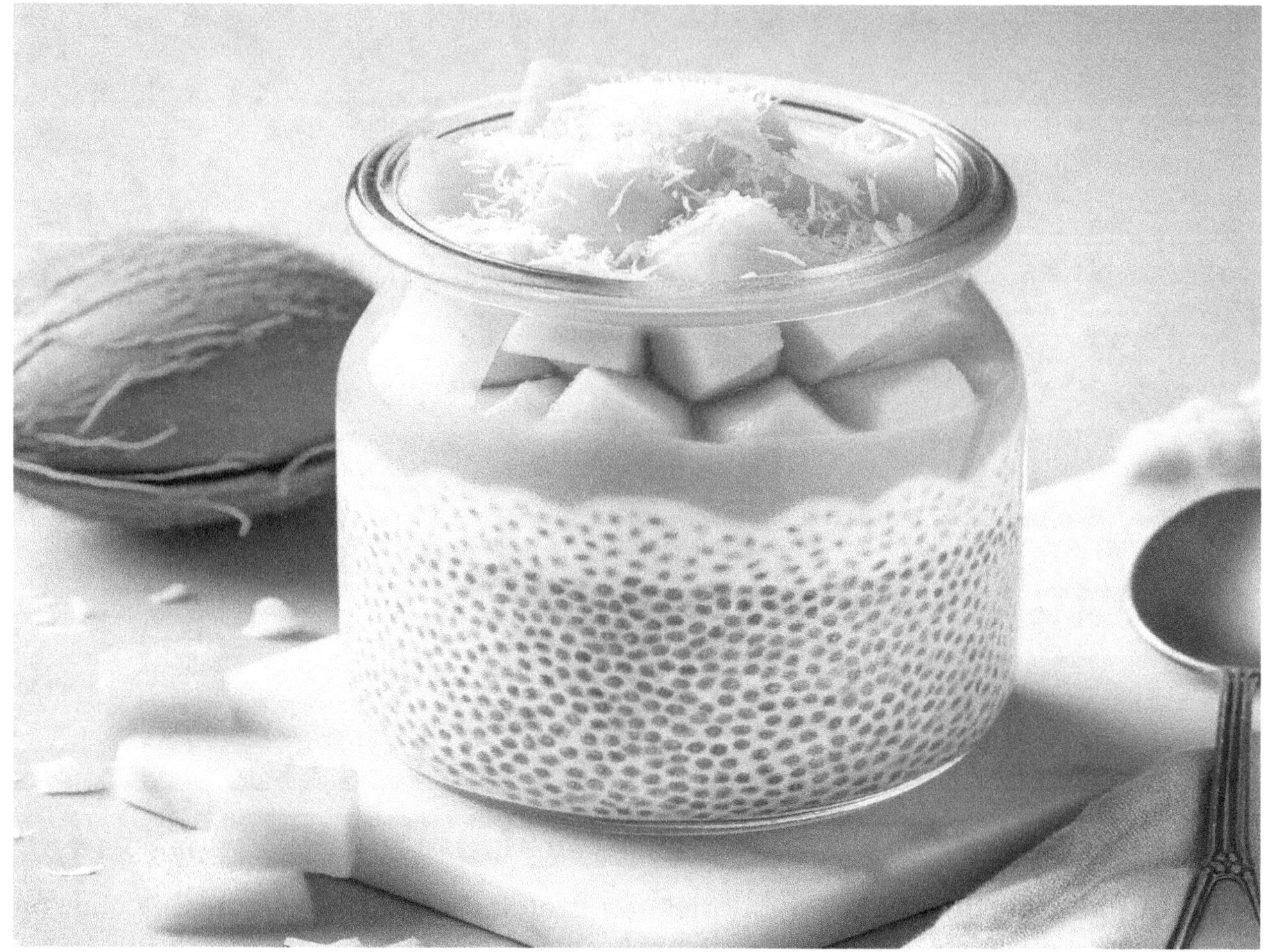

Mango Chia Pudding

Nutritional Information: 340 calories, 5g protein, 30g carbohydrates, 24g fat, 11g fiber, 45mg sodium.

Ingredients:

- 1/4 cup chia seeds
- 1 cup coconut milk
- 1/2 cup mango puree
- 1 tablespoon coconut flakes

Prep Time: 10 minutes (plus chilling), **Cook Time**: 0 minutes, **Servings**: 1

Instructions:

1. In a jar, mix the chia seeds with coconut milk. Let sit for at least 30 minutes or overnight in the refrigerator until the mixture achieves a pudding-like consistency.

2. Layer the mango puree over the chia pudding.

3. Top with coconut flakes before serving.

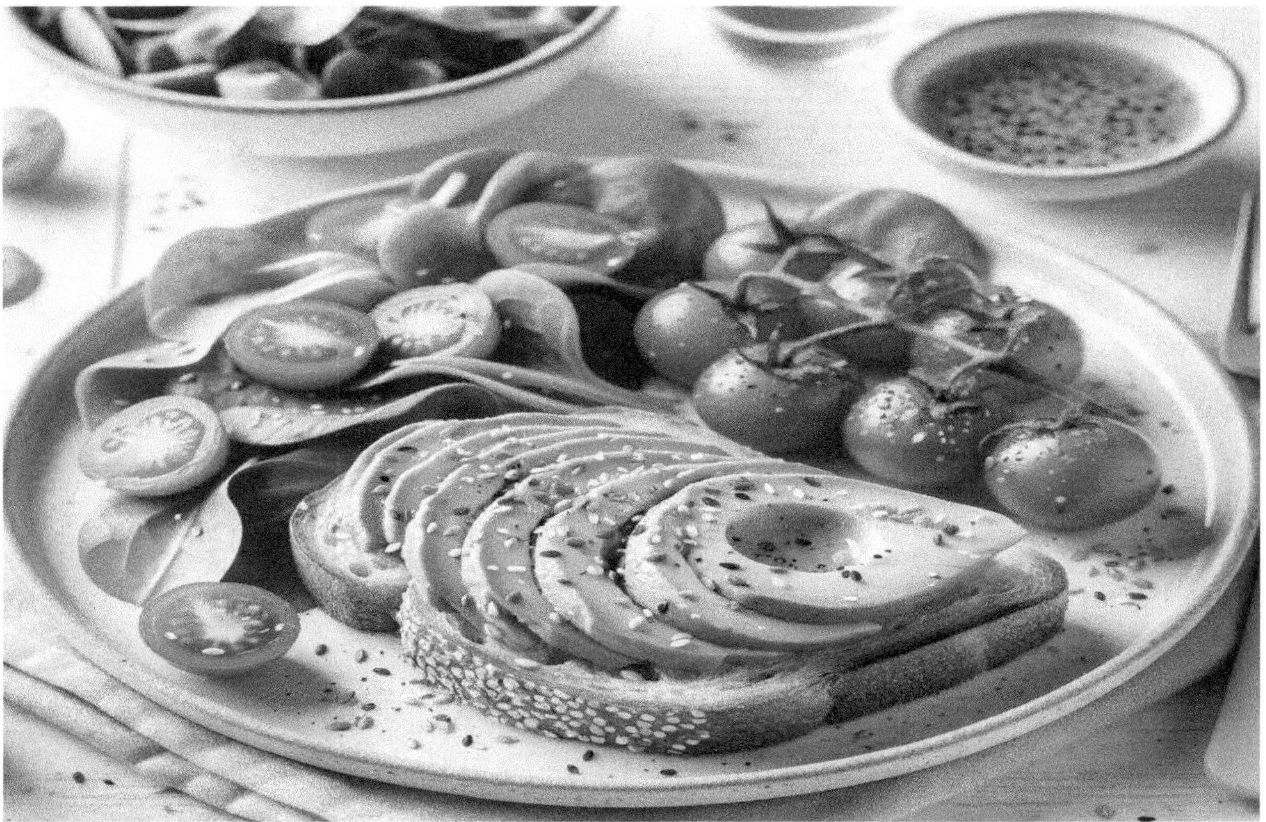

Avocado Toast with Cherry Tomatoes

Nutritional Information: 250 calories, 6g protein, 27g carbohydrates, 15g fat, 9g fiber, 180mg sodium.

Ingredients:

- 1 slice whole grain bread
- 1/2 avocado, mashed
- 5 cherry tomatoes, halved
- 1 teaspoon sesame seeds
- Salt and pepper to taste

Prep Time: 5 minutes, **Cook Time**: 2 minutes, **Servings**: 1

Instructions:

1. Toast the whole grain bread to your liking.

2. Spread the mashed avocado evenly on the toast.

3. Top with halved cherry tomatoes and sprinkle with sesame seeds.

4. Season with salt and pepper to taste and serve.

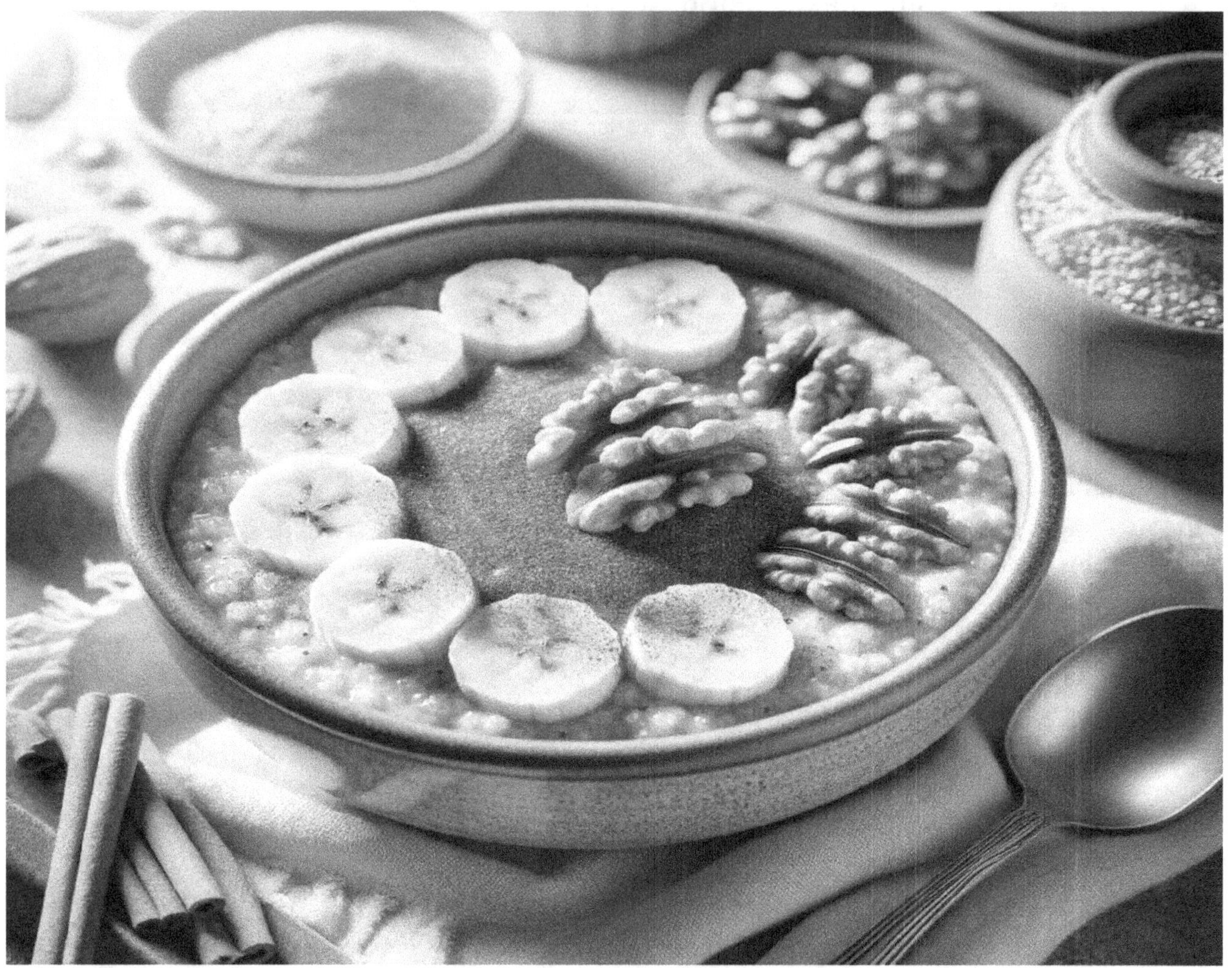

Quinoa Banana Nut Porridge

Nutritional Information: 320 calories, 9g protein, 53g carbohydrates, 7g fat, 6g fiber, 30mg sodium.

Ingredients:

- 1/2 cup quinoa, rinsed
- 1 cup almond milk
- 1 banana, sliced
- 1 tablespoon walnuts, chopped
- 1/2 teaspoon cinnamon

Prep Time: 5 minutes, **Cook Time**: 15 minutes, **Servings**: 1

Instructions:

1. Combine quinoa and almond milk in a small saucepan and bring to a boil.

2. Reduce heat to low, cover, and simmer for 15 minutes or until quinoa is cooked and most of the liquid is absorbed.

3. Remove from heat and let it sit covered for 5 minutes.

4. Stir in sliced bananas, walnuts, and cinnamon.

5. Serve warm for a comforting and nutritious start to your day.

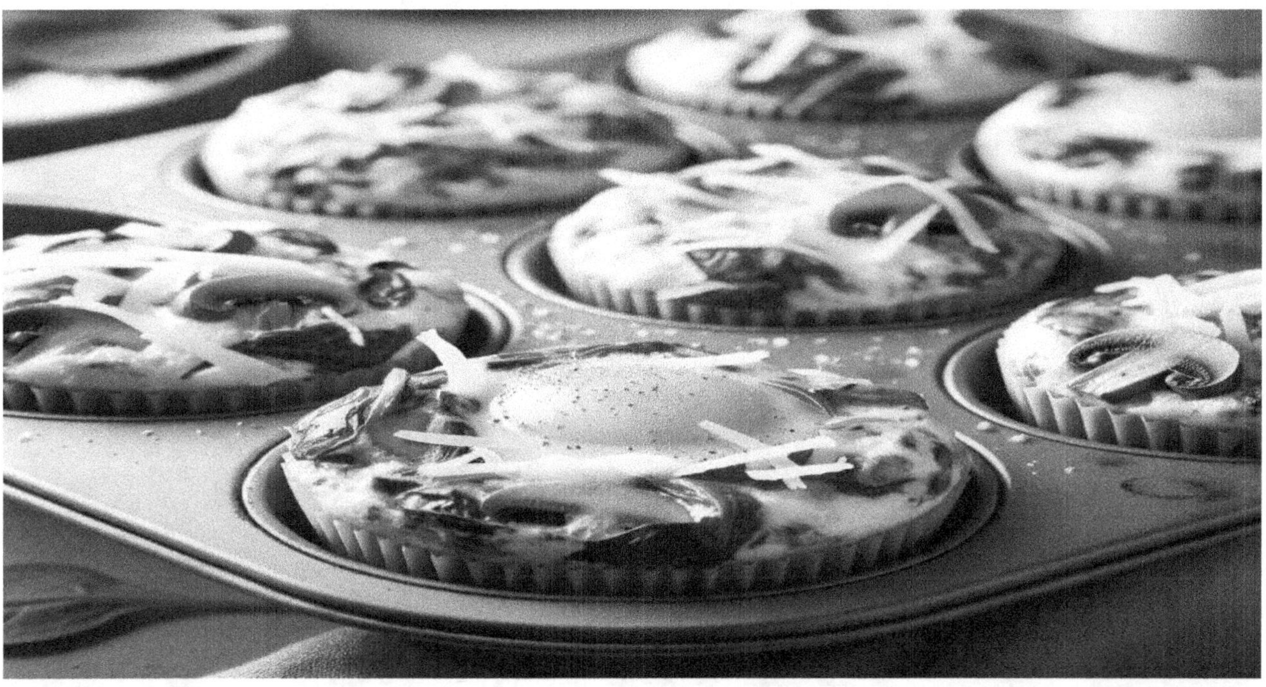

Spinach and Mushroom Egg Muffins

Nutritional Information: Calories: 100, Protein: 8g, Carbohydrates: 3g, Fat: 6g, Fiber: 1g, Sodium: 125mg.

Ingredients:

- 6 eggs
- 1 cup fresh spinach, chopped
- 1/2 cup mushrooms, chopped
- 1/4 cup onions, finely chopped
- 1/4 cup shredded low-fat cheese
- Salt and pepper to taste

Prep Time: 10 minutes, **Cook Time**: 20 minutes, **Servings**: 6

Instructions:

1. Preheat oven to 375°F (190°C). Grease a muffin tin or line with paper liners.

2. In a bowl, beat the eggs. Add spinach, mushrooms, onions, cheese, salt, and pepper.

3. Pour the egg mixture evenly into the muffin tins.

4. Bake for 20 minutes, or until the egg muffins are firm and golden on top.

5. Let cool for a few minutes before serving.

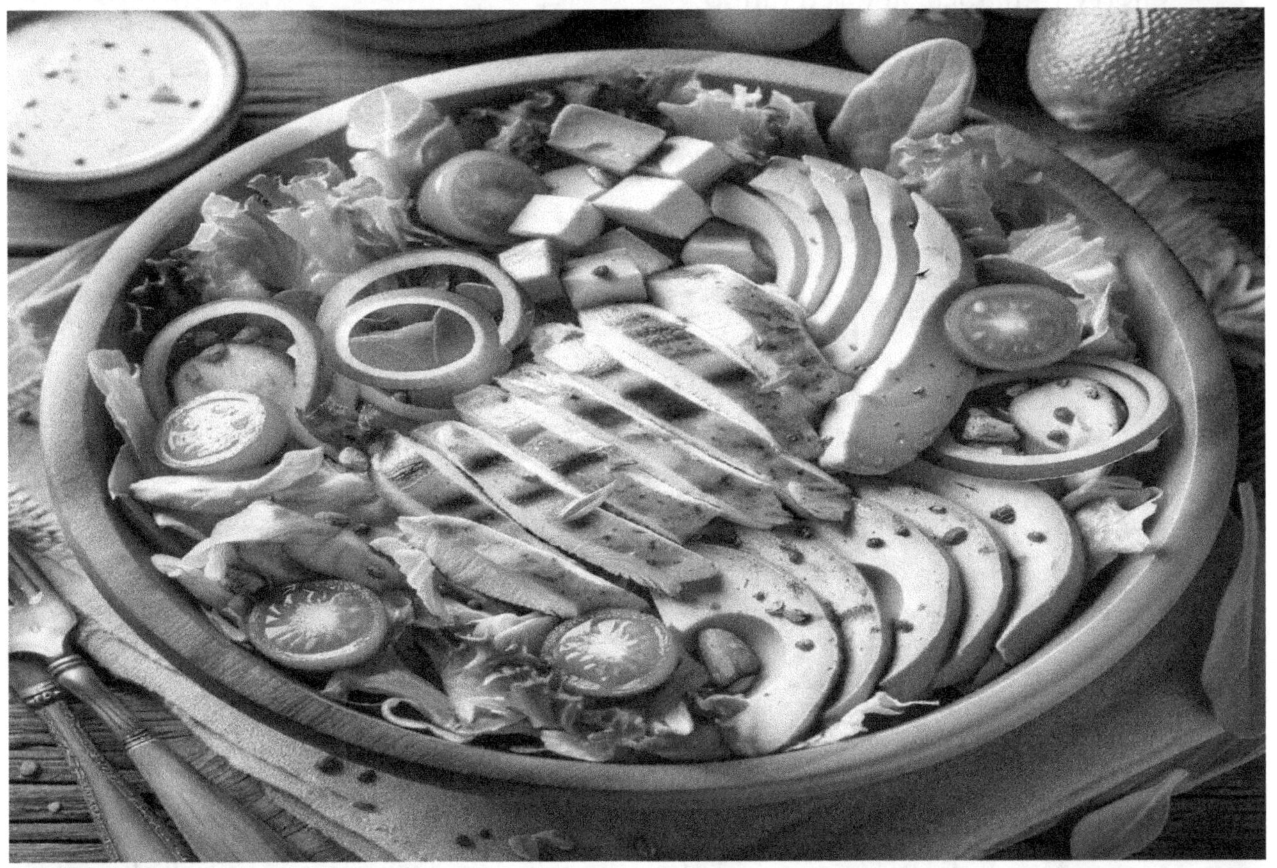

Grilled Chicken and Avocado Salad

Nutritional Information: 370 calories, 26g protein, 14g carbohydrates, 22g fat, 6g fiber, 180mg sodium.

Ingredients:

- 2 boneless, skinless chicken breasts, grilled and sliced
- 2 cups mixed greens
- 1 avocado, sliced
- 1/2 cup cherry tomatoes, halved
- 1/4 red onion, thinly sliced
- 2 tablespoons olive oil
- 1 tablespoon lemon juice
- Salt and pepper to taste

Prep Time: 10 minutes, **Cook Time**: 10 minutes, **Servings**: 2

Instructions:

1. Arrange mixed greens on a plate. Top with sliced grilled chicken, avocado, cherry tomatoes, and red onion.

2. In a small bowl, whisk together olive oil, lemon juice, salt, and pepper.

3. Drizzle the dressing over the salad and serve.

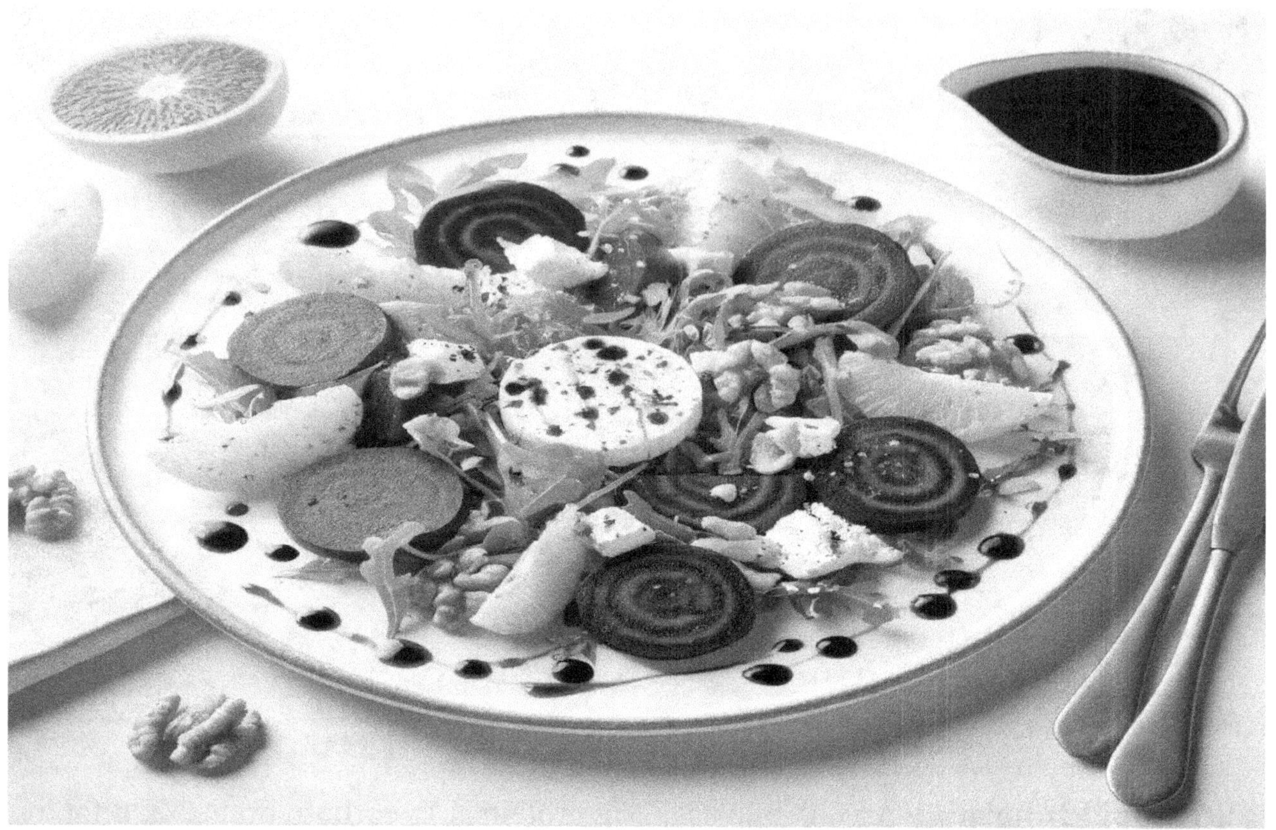

Beetroot and Goat Cheese Salad

Nutritional Information: 295 calories, 9g protein, 21g carbohydrates, 19g fat, 5g fiber, 220mg sodium.

Ingredients:

- 2 medium beetroots, cooked and sliced
- 1/2 cup goat cheese, crumbled
- 2 cups arugula
- 1/4 cup walnuts, chopped
- 1 orange, peeled and segments
- 2 tablespoons balsamic reduction
- Salt and pepper to taste

Prep Time: 15 minutes, **Cook Time**: 0 minutes, **Servings**: 2

1. Place arugula on a plate and arrange beetroot slices and orange segments on top.

2. Sprinkle with crumbled goat cheese and chopped walnuts.

3. Drizzle with balsamic reduction and season with salt and pepper to serve.

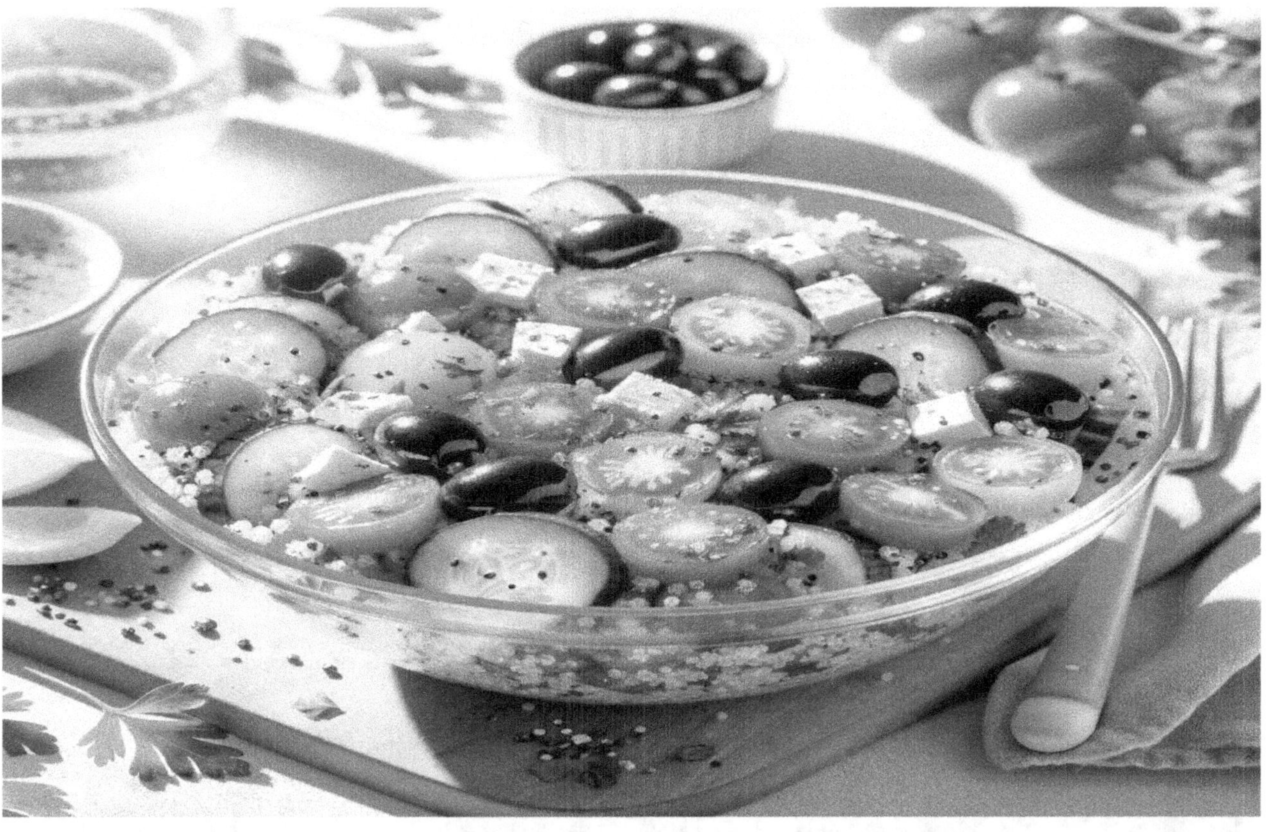

Mediterranean Quinoa Salad

Nutritional Information: 320 calories, 8g protein, 30g carbohydrates, 18g fat, 5g fiber, 320mg sodium.

Ingredients:

- 1 cup cooked quinoa
- 1/2 cup cherry tomatoes, halved
- 1/2 cucumber, diced
- 1/4 cup black olives, sliced
- 1/4 cup feta cheese, crumbled
- 2 tablespoons parsley, chopped
- 2 tablespoons olive oil
- 1 tablespoon lemon juice
- Salt and pepper to taste

Prep Time: 15 minutes, **Cook Time**: 15 minutes, **Servings**: 2

Instructions:

1. In a large bowl, combine cooked quinoa, cherry tomatoes, cucumber, black olives, and feta cheese.

2. Add parsley, olive oil, and lemon juice. Toss to combine.

3. Season with salt and pepper and serve chilled.

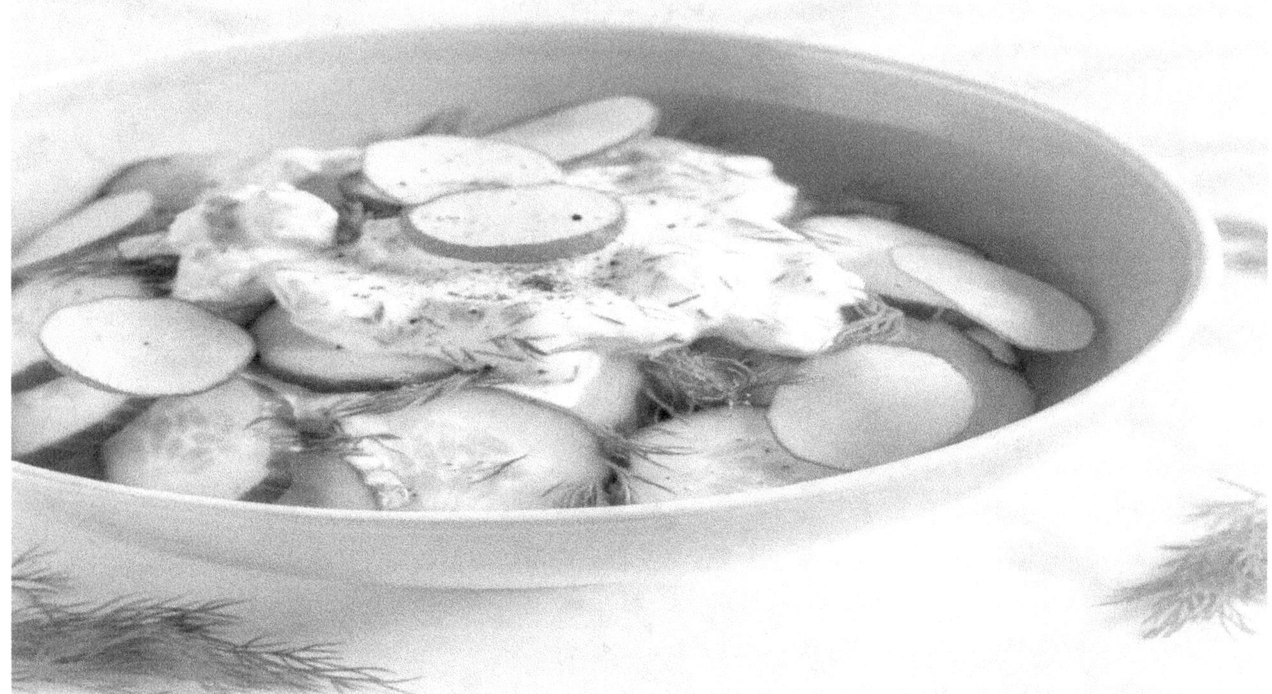

Cucumber and Dill Salad

Nutritional Information: 90 calories, 3g protein, 12g carbohydrates, 3g fat, 2g fiber, 50mg sodium.

Ingredients:

- 2 large cucumbers, sliced
- 1/4 cup Greek yogurt
- 2 tablespoons fresh dill, chopped
- 1 tablespoon lemon juice
- 1/4 teaspoon garlic powder
- Salt and pepper to taste
- 4 radishes, thinly sliced

Prep Time: 10 minutes, **Cook Time**: 0 minutes, **Servings**: 2

1. In a bowl, mix Greek yogurt, dill, lemon juice, garlic powder, salt, and pepper to create the dressing.

2. Add cucumber and radish slices to the bowl and toss well to coat.

3. Chill for about 10 minutes before serving to let flavors meld.

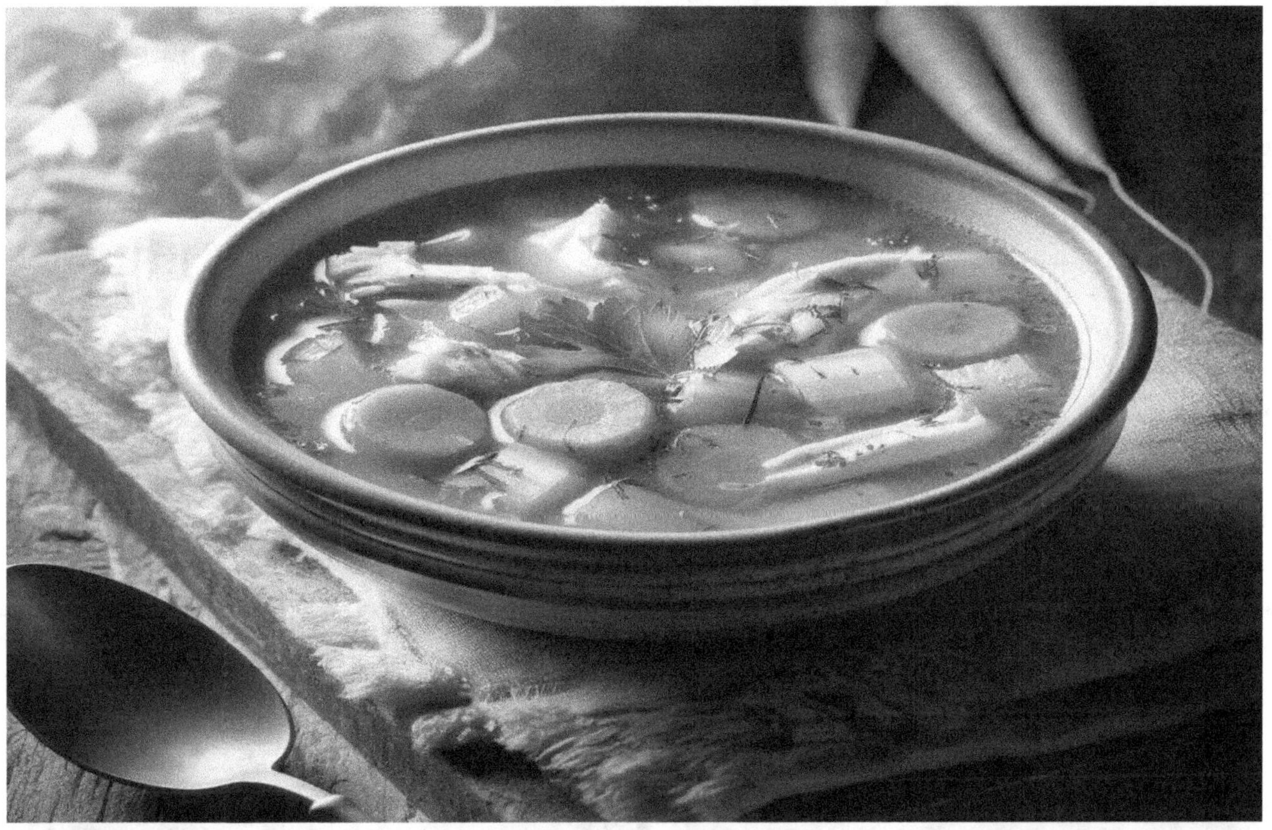

Chicken and Vegetable Soup

Nutritional Information: Calories: 165, Protein: 25g, Carbohydrates: 8g, Fat: 3g, Fiber: 2g, Sodium: 420mg.

Ingredients:

- 2 boneless, skinless chicken breasts, diced
- 1 cup carrots, diced
- 1 cup celery, diced
- 1 onion, chopped
- 2 cloves garlic, minced
- 6 cups low-sodium chicken broth
- 1 teaspoon dried thyme
- 1 teaspoon dried parsley

- Salt and pepper to taste

Prep Time: 10 minutes, **Cook Time**: 20 minutes, **Servings**: 4

Instructions:

1. In a large pot, sauté onions and garlic until translucent.
2. Add chicken and cook until browned.
3. Add carrots, celery, thyme, and parsley. Pour in chicken broth and bring to a boil.
4. Reduce heat and simmer for 20 minutes or until vegetables are tender.
5. Season with salt and pepper. Serve hot.

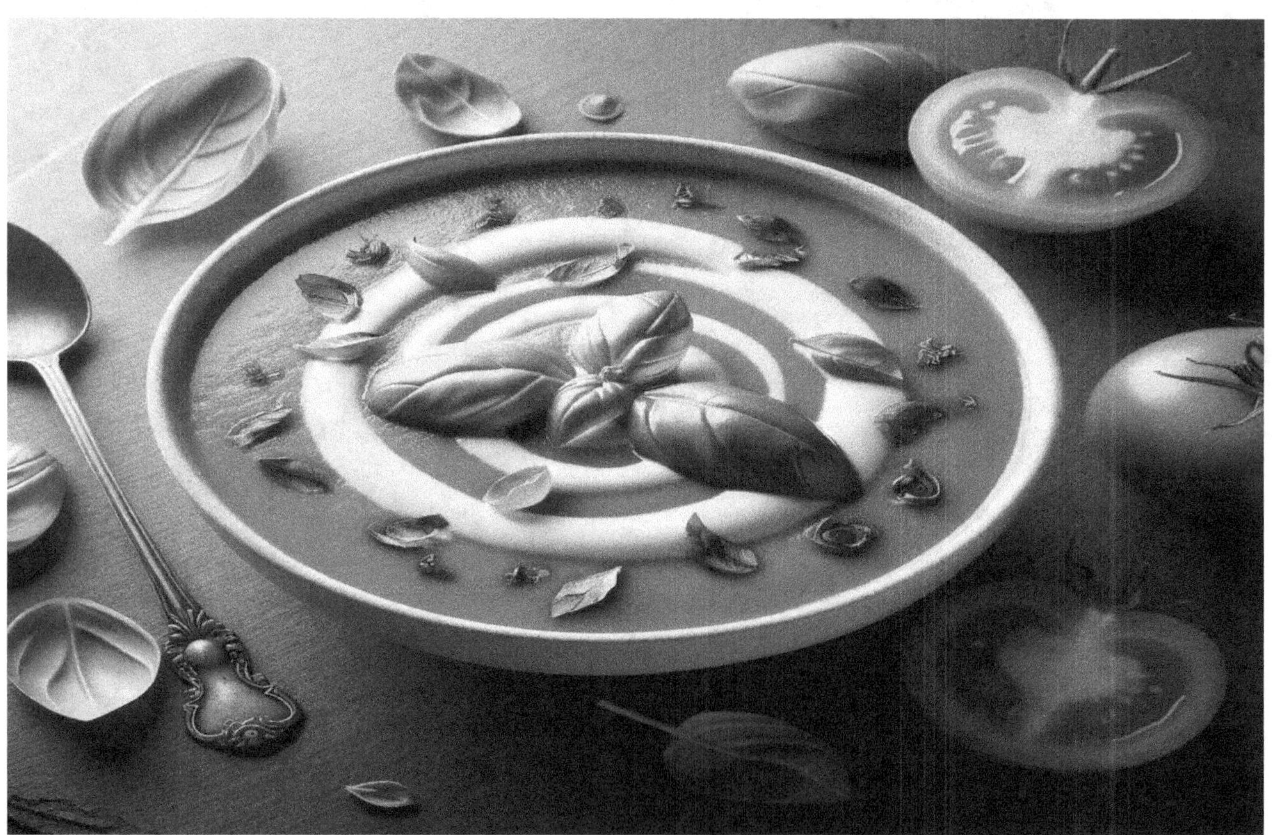

Creamy Tomato Basil Soup

Nutritional Information: Calories: 140, Protein: 3g, Carbohydrates: 15g, Fat: 8g, Fiber: 3g, Sodium: 280mg.

Ingredients:

- 4 cups chopped tomatoes
- 1 onion, chopped

- 2 cloves garlic, minced
- 2 cups vegetable broth
- 1/2 cup low-fat cream
- 1/4 cup fresh basil, chopped
- Salt and pepper to taste

Prep Time: 5 minutes, **Cook Time**: 15 minutes, **Servings**: 4

Instructions:

1. In a pot, sauté onion and garlic until soft.
2. Add tomatoes and vegetable broth, bring to a boil, then simmer for 10 minutes.
3. Blend the soup until smooth, return to the pot.
4. Stir in cream and basil, heat through.
5. Season with salt and pepper, serve warm.

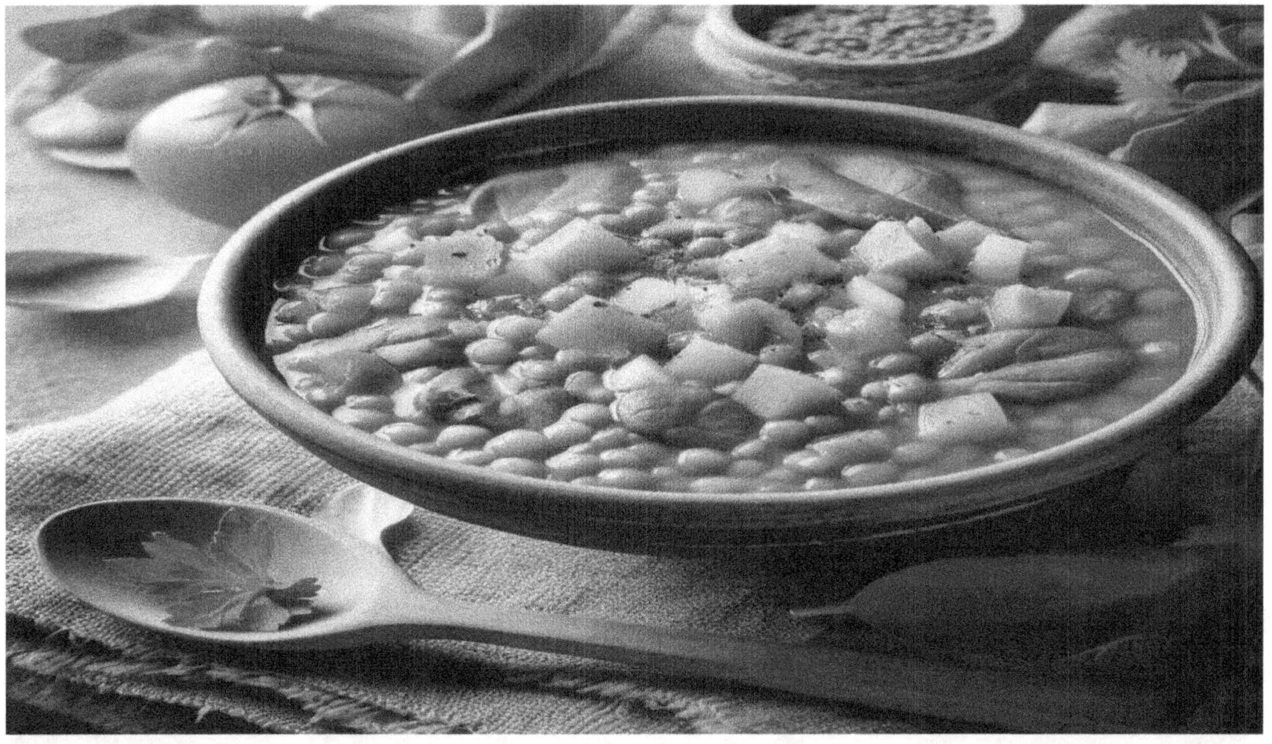

Lentil Vegetable Soup

Nutritional Information: Calories: 180, Protein: 12g, Carbohydrates: 30g, Fat: 2g, Fiber: 8g, Sodium: 300mg.

Ingredients:

- 1 cup dry lentils, rinsed
- 1 carrot, diced

- 1 stalk celery, diced
- 1 onion, diced
- 2 cloves garlic, minced
- 1 tomato, chopped
- 6 cups vegetable broth
-

- 1 teaspoon cumin
- 1/2 teaspoon coriander
- Salt and pepper to taste
- Fresh parsley, chopped for garnish

Prep Time: 10 minutes, **Cook Time**: 30 minutes, **Servings**: 4

Instructions:

1. In a large pot, sauté onions, garlic, carrots, and celery until soft.
2. Add lentils, tomatoes, cumin, and coriander. Pour in vegetable broth and bring to a boil.
3. Reduce heat and simmer for 25 minutes or until lentils are tender.
4. Season with salt and pepper. Garnish with fresh parsley before serving.

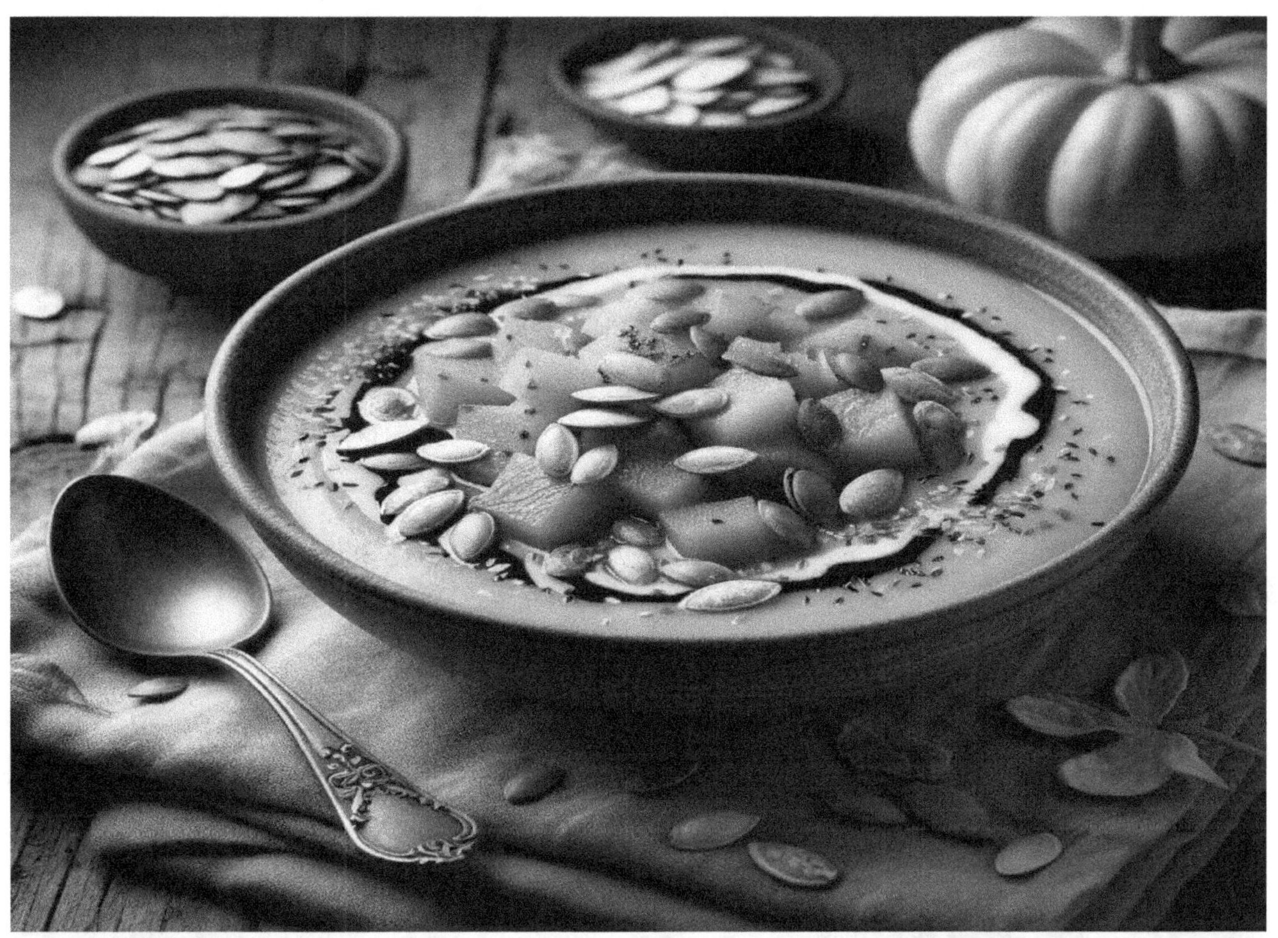

Spicy Butternut Squash Soup

Nutritional Information: Calories: 175, Protein: 3g, Carbohydrates: 30g, Fat: 5g, Fiber: 6g, Sodium: 250mg.

Ingredients:

- 1 medium butternut squash, peeled and cubed
- 1 onion, chopped
- 2 cloves garlic, minced
- 4 cups vegetable broth
- 1 teaspoon chili powder
- 1/2 teaspoon smoked paprika
- 1/4 cup coconut milk
- Roasted pumpkin seeds for garnish

Prep Time: 15 minutes, **Cook Time**: 25 minutes, **Servings**: 4

Instructions:

1. In a large pot, sauté onion and garlic until translucent.

2. Add butternut squash, vegetable broth, chili powder, and paprika. Bring to a boil, then simmer until squash is tender.

3. Blend the soup until smooth. Stir in coconut milk and heat through.

4. Serve hot, garnished with roasted pumpkin seeds.

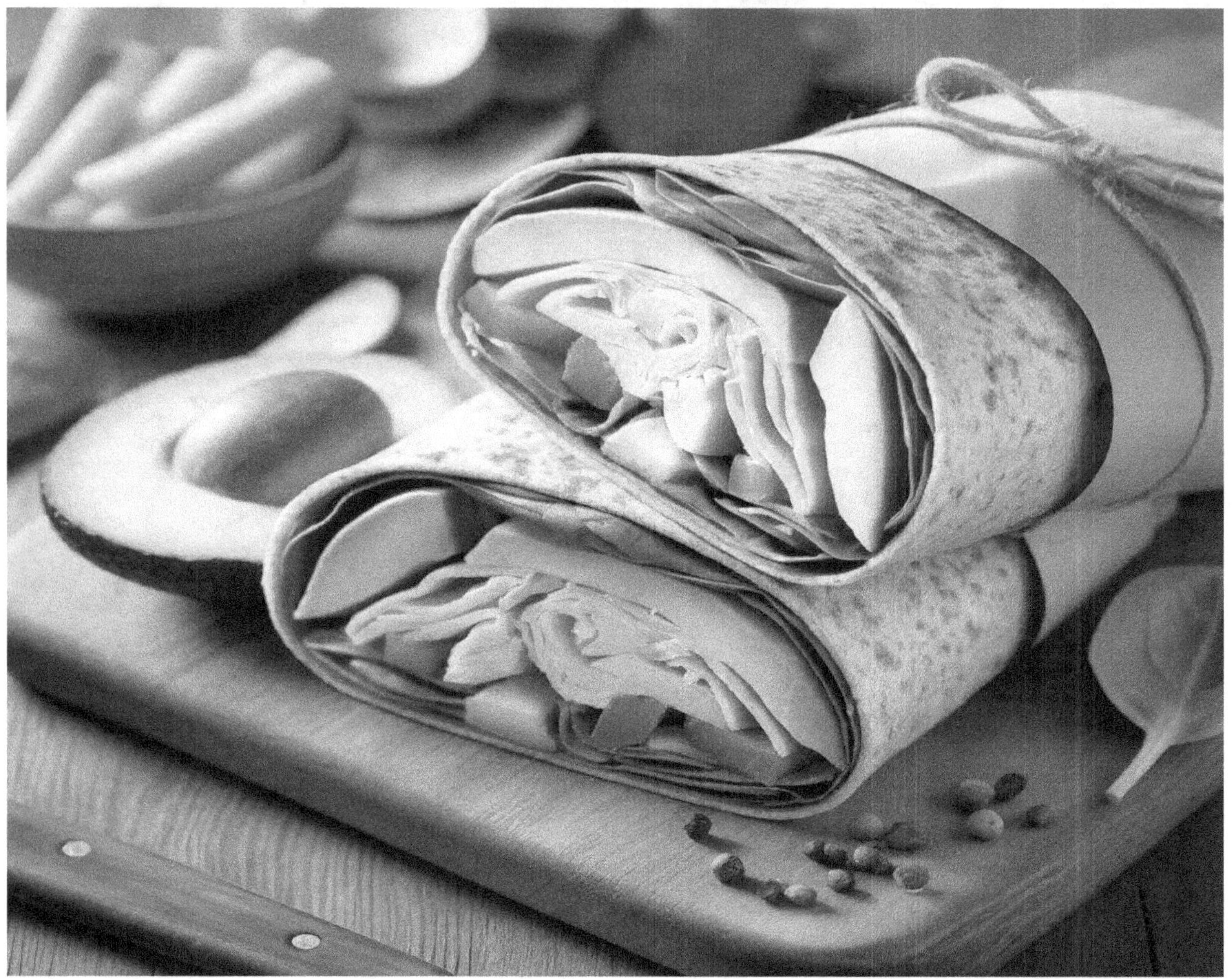

Turkey and Avocado Wrap

Nutritional Information: Calories: 350, Protein: 25g, Carbohydrates: 27g, Fat: 17g, Fiber: 6g, Sodium: 420mg.

Ingredients:

- 1 whole grain tortilla
- 3 ounces sliced turkey breast
- 1/2 ripe avocado, sliced

- 1/2 cup spinach leaves
- 2 tablespoons shredded carrot
- 1 tablespoon hummus

Prep Time: 5 minutes, **Cook Time**: 0 minutes, **Servings**: 1

Instructions:

1. Spread hummus evenly over the tortilla.

2. Layer turkey slices, avocado, spinach, and carrots on top.

3. Roll the tortilla tightly, cut in half, and serve.

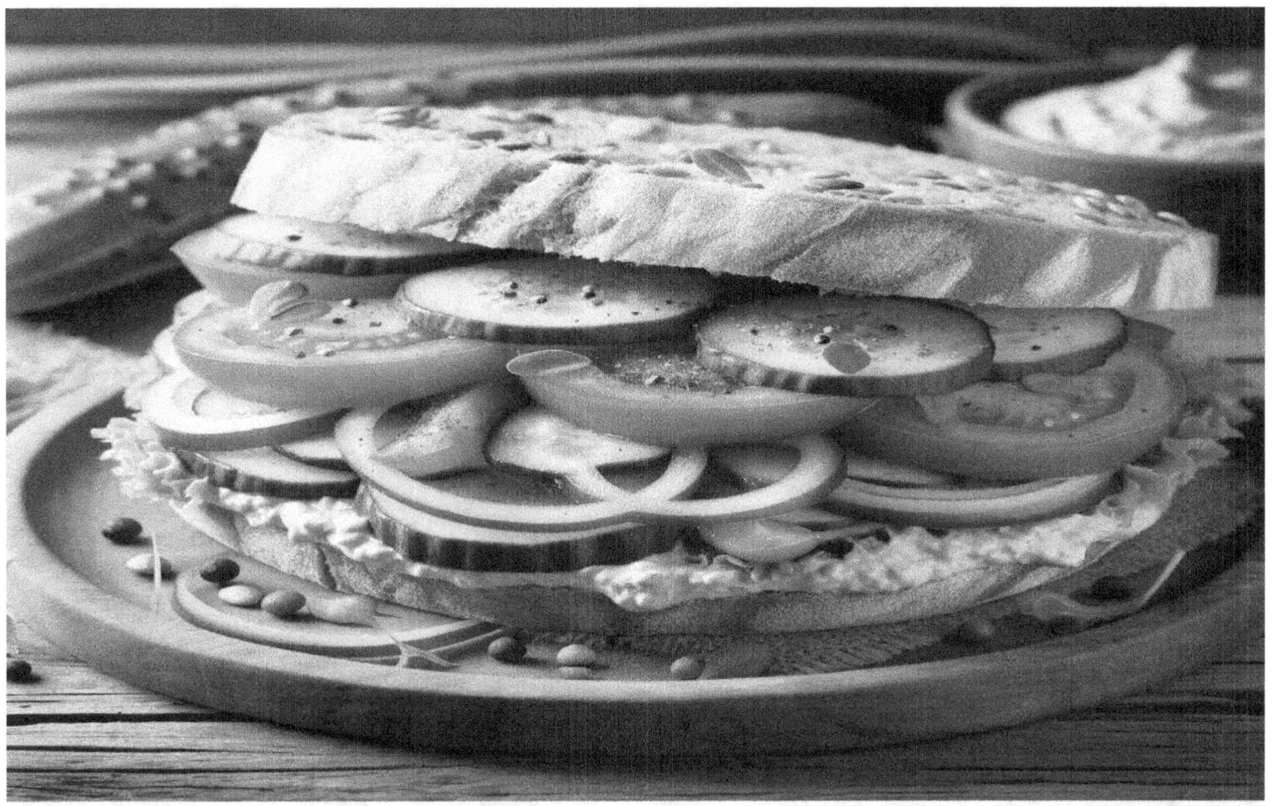

Mediterranean Veggie Sandwich

Nutritional Information: Calories: 320, Protein: 12g, Carbohydrates: 45g, Fat: 12g, Fiber: 7g, Sodium: 560mg.

Ingredients:

- 2 slices whole grain bread
- 2 tablespoons hummus
- 1/4 cucumber, sliced
- 2 slices tomato
- 2 slices red onion
- 1/4 cup mixed greens
- 1 tablespoon feta cheese, crumbled

Prep Time: 10 minutes, **Cook Time**: 0 minutes, **Servings**: 1

Instructions:

1. Spread hummus on both slices of bread.

2. Layer cucumber, tomato, onion, and greens on one slice.

3. Sprinkle feta cheese over the vegetables.

4. Top with the second slice of bread, cut in half, and serve.

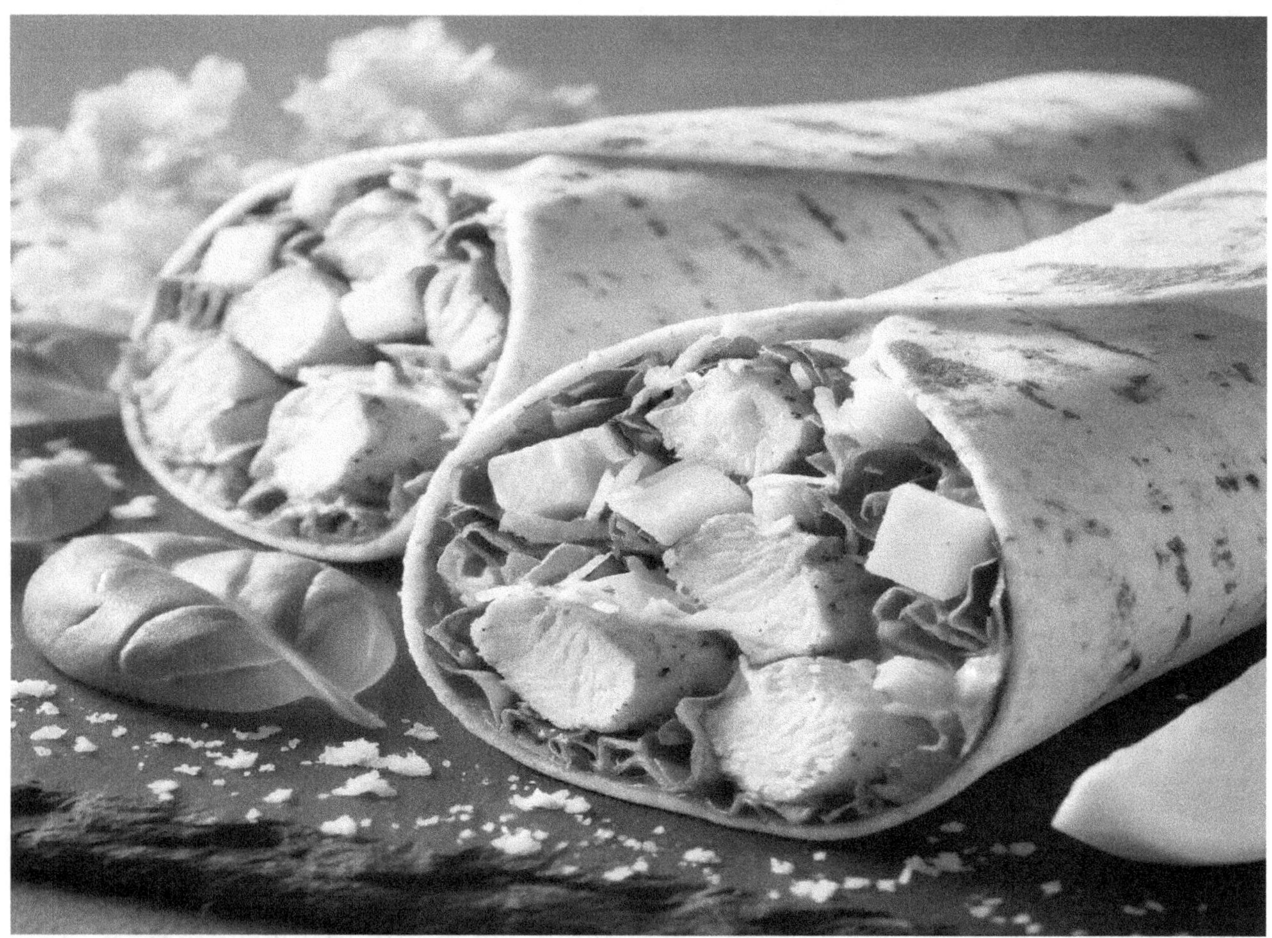

Grilled Chicken Caesar Wrap

Nutritional Information: Calories: 380, Protein: 28g, Carbohydrates: 32g, Fat: 16g, Fiber: 5g, Sodium: 690mg.

Ingredients:

- 1 whole grain tortilla

- 3 ounces grilled chicken breast, sliced

- 1 cup romaine lettuce, chopped

- 2 tablespoons Caesar dressing, low-fat

- 1 tablespoon grated Parmesan cheese

-

- 1 teaspoon lemon juice

Prep Time: 10 minutes, **Cook Time**: 10 minutes, **Servings**: 1

Instructions:

1. Toss chicken, lettuce, Caesar dressing, and lemon juice in a bowl.

2. Sprinkle Parmesan cheese over the mixture.

3. Place the filling on the tortilla, roll tightly, slice in half, and serve.

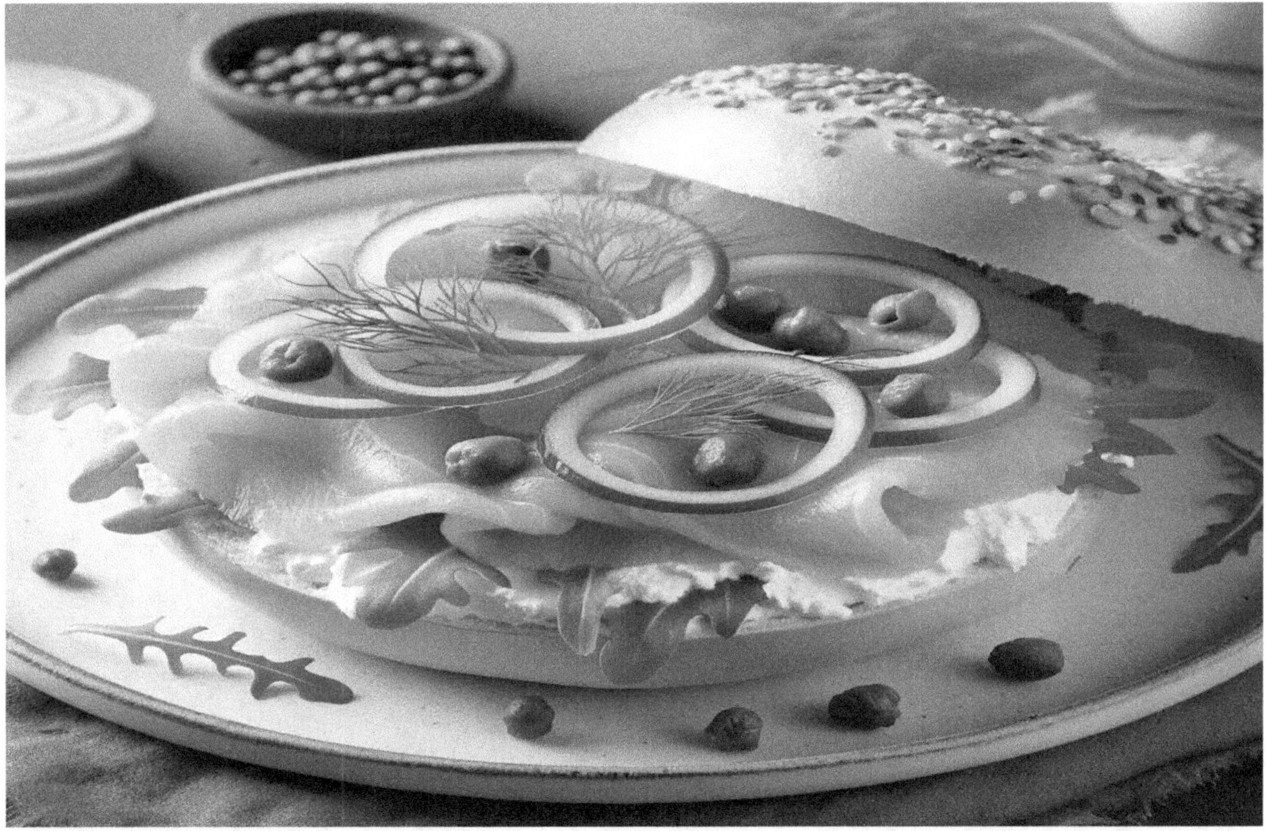

Smoked Salmon and Cream Cheese Bagel

Nutritional Information: Calories: 400, Protein: 23g, Carbohydrates: 53g, Fat: 12g, Fiber: 8g, Sodium: 580mg.

Ingredients:

- 1 whole grain bagel, halved

- 2 ounces smoked salmon

- 2 tablespoons light cream cheese

- 1/4 cup arugula
- 2 slices red onion
- 1 tablespoon capers
- 1 teaspoon fresh dill

Prep Time: 5 minutes, **Cook Time**: 0 minute, **Servings**: 1

Instructions:

1. Spread cream cheese on each half of the bagel.

2. Layer smoked salmon, arugula, onion, and capers on one half.

3. Sprinkle dill over the top, cover with the other half, and serve.

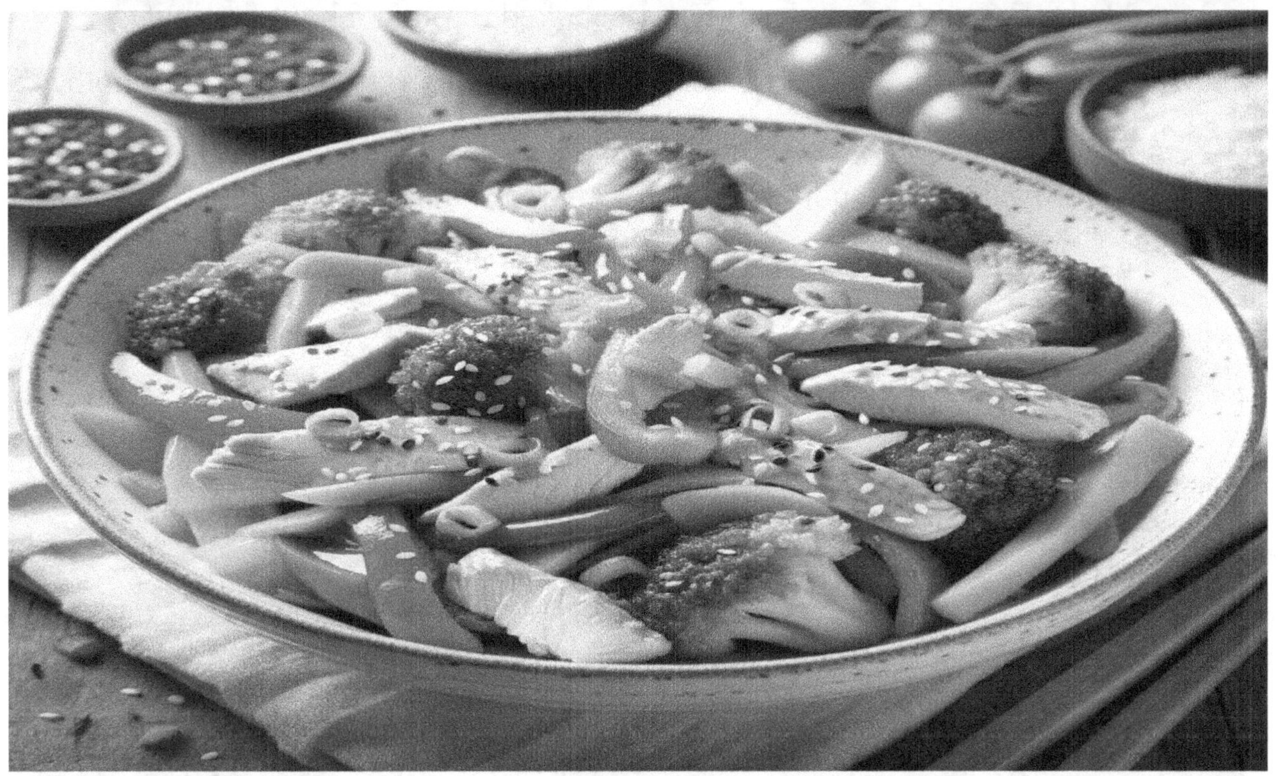

Chicken and Vegetable Stir-Fry

Nutritional Information: Calories: 295, Protein: 34g, Carbohydrates: 15g, Fat: 11g, Fiber: 3g, Sodium: 430mg.

Ingredients:

- 2 boneless, skinless chicken breasts, thinly sliced
- 1 cup broccoli florets
- 1/2 red bell pepper, sliced
- 1/2 yellow bell pepper, sliced
- 1/2 cup carrots, julienned
- 2 tablespoons low-sodium soy sauce
- 1 tablespoon sesame oil
- 1 teaspoon honey
- 1 garlic clove, minced
- 1 teaspoon grated ginger
- Sesame seeds and sliced green onions for garnish

Prep Time: 10 minutes, **Cook Time**: 10 minutes, **Servings**: 2

Instructions:

1. Heat sesame oil in a large skillet over medium-high heat.

2. Add chicken and stir-fry until nearly cooked through, about 5 minutes.

3. Add garlic, ginger, broccoli, bell peppers, and carrots. Stir-fry for another 5 minutes.

4. Stir in soy sauce and honey, cook for an additional 2 minutes.

5. Garnish with sesame seeds and green onions before serving.

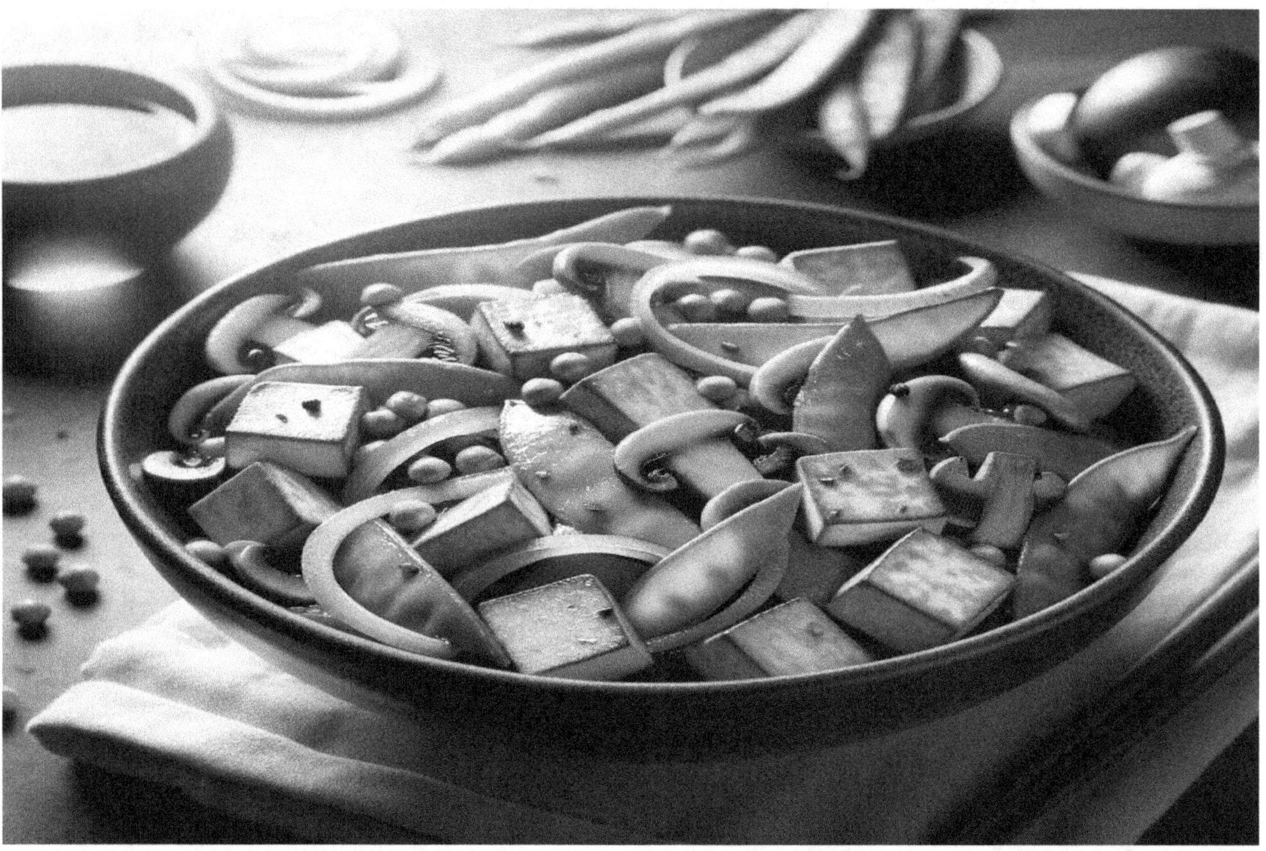

Tofu and Snap Pea Stir-Fry

Nutritional Information: Calories: 250, Protein: 18g, Carbohydrates: 15g, Fat: 14g, Fiber: 4g, Sodium: 330mg.

Ingredients:

- 1 block firm tofu, drained and cubed
- 1 cup snap peas
- 1/2 cup mushrooms, sliced
- 1 red onion, sliced
- 2 tablespoons low-sodium soy sauce
- 1 tablespoon olive oil

- 1 teaspoon sesame seeds

Prep Time: 10 minutes, **Cook Time**: 10 minutes, **Servings**: 2

Instructions:

1. Heat olive oil in a skillet over medium-high heat.

2. Add tofu and stir-fry until golden brown, about 5 minutes.

3. Add snap peas, mushrooms, and red onion, and stir-fry for another 5 minutes.

4. Drizzle with soy sauce and sprinkle with sesame seeds before serving.

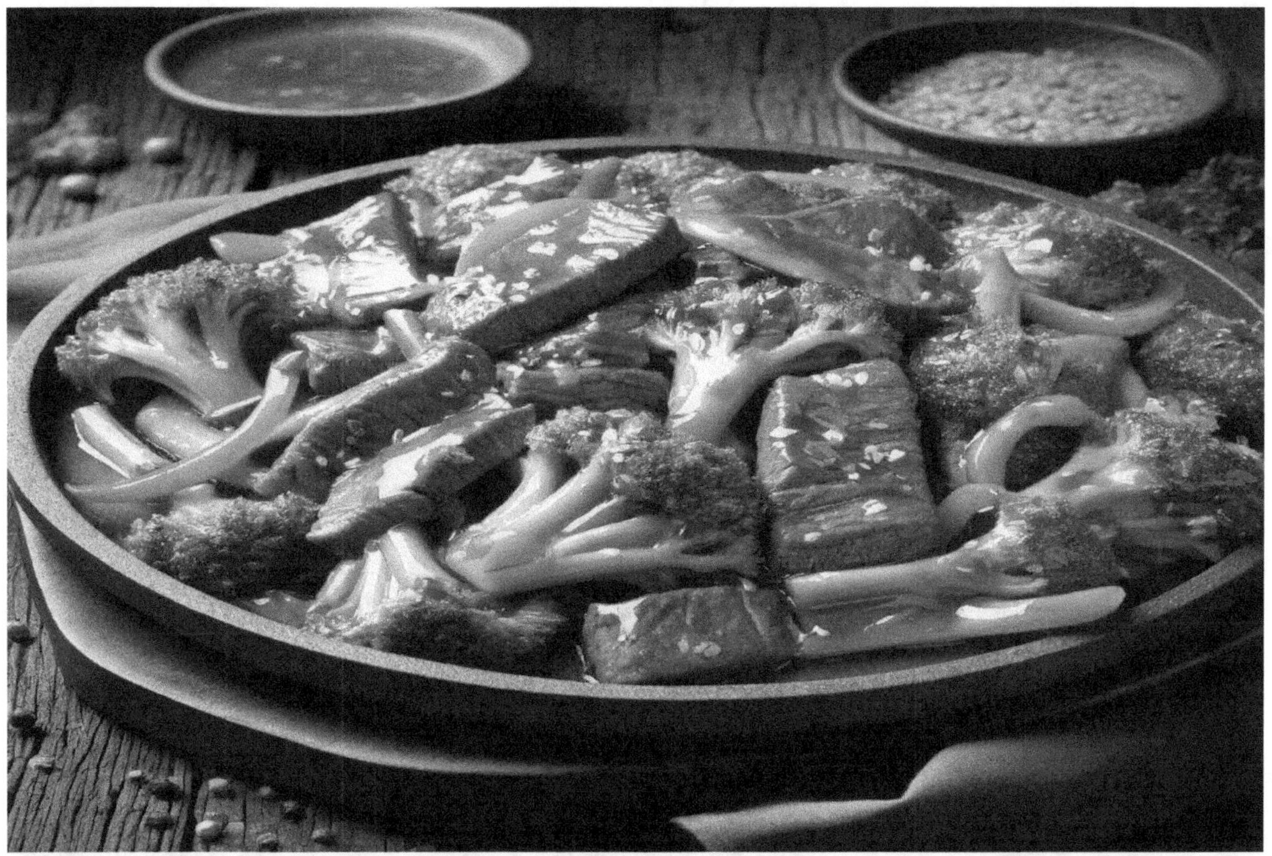

Beef and Broccoli Stir-Fry

Nutritional Information: Calories: 275, Protein: 26g, Carbohydrates: 10g, Fat: 15g, Fiber: 3g, Sodium: 400mg.

Ingredients:

- 8 oz lean beef, thinly sliced

- 2 cups broccoli florets

- 1/2 bell pepper, sliced

- 2 tablespoons oyster sauce

- 1 tablespoon vegetable oil
- 1 garlic clove, minced
- 1 teaspoon grated ginger

Prep Time: 10 minutes, **Cook Time**: 10 minutes, **Servings**: 2

Instructions:

1. Heat oil in a pan over high heat.

2. Add beef and stir-fry until it starts to brown, about 3 minutes.

3. Add garlic, ginger, broccoli, and bell pepper. Continue to stir-fry for about 5 minutes.

4. Stir in oyster sauce and cook for another 2 minutes until everything is well coated and cooked through.

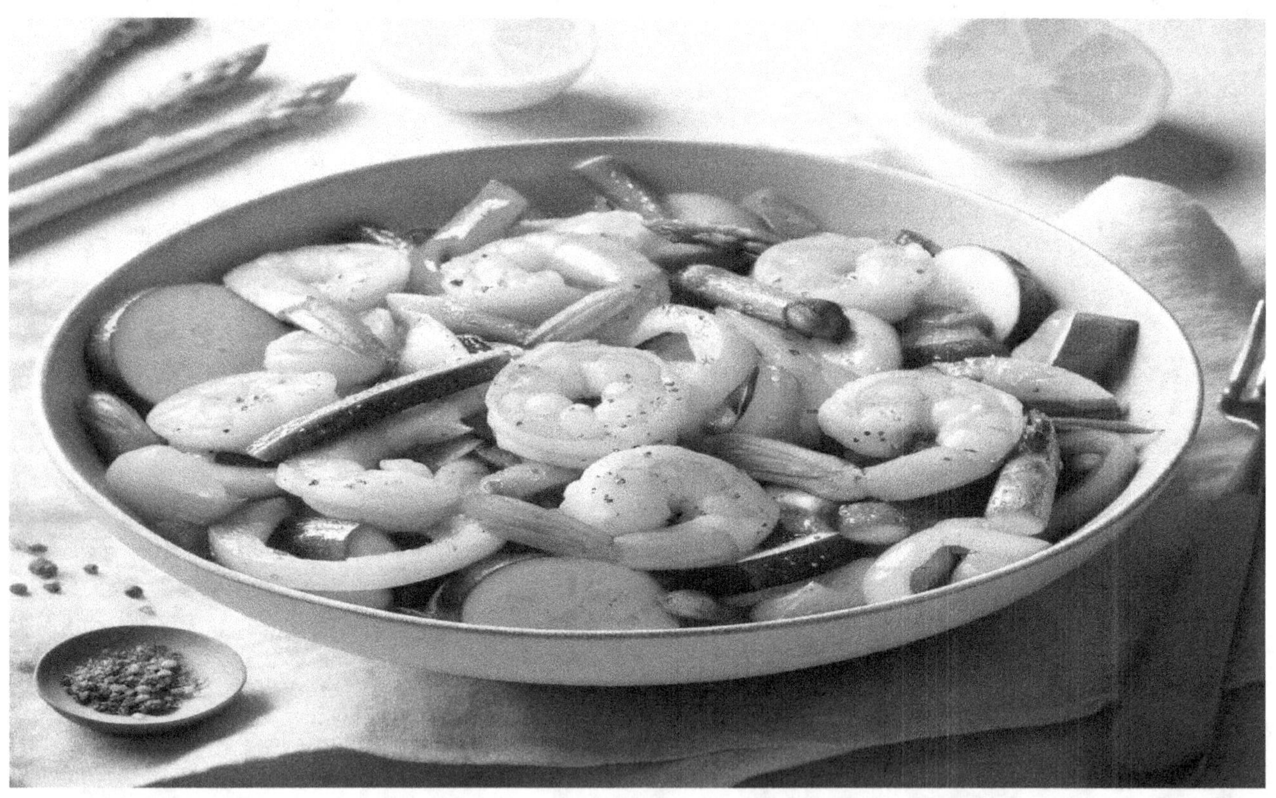

Shrimp and Bell Pepper Stir-Fry

Nutritional Information: Calories: 210, Protein: 24g, Carbohydrates: 12g, Fat: 8g, Fiber: 3g, Sodium: 285mg.

Ingredients:

- 8 oz shrimp, peeled and deveined
- 1/2 cup red bell pepper, sliced
- 1/2 cup yellow bell pepper, sliced
- 1/2 cup zucchini, sliced
- 1/2 cup asparagus, chopped
- 2 tablespoons lemon juice
- 1 tablespoon olive oil
- Salt and pepper to taste

Prep Time: 10 minutes, **Cook Time**: 8 minutes, **Servings**: 2

Instructions:

1. Heat olive oil in a skillet over medium-high heat.
2. Add shrimp and vegetables, stir-fry until shrimp are pink and vegetables are tender, about 6-8 minutes.
3. Drizzle with lemon juice, season with salt and pepper, and serve.

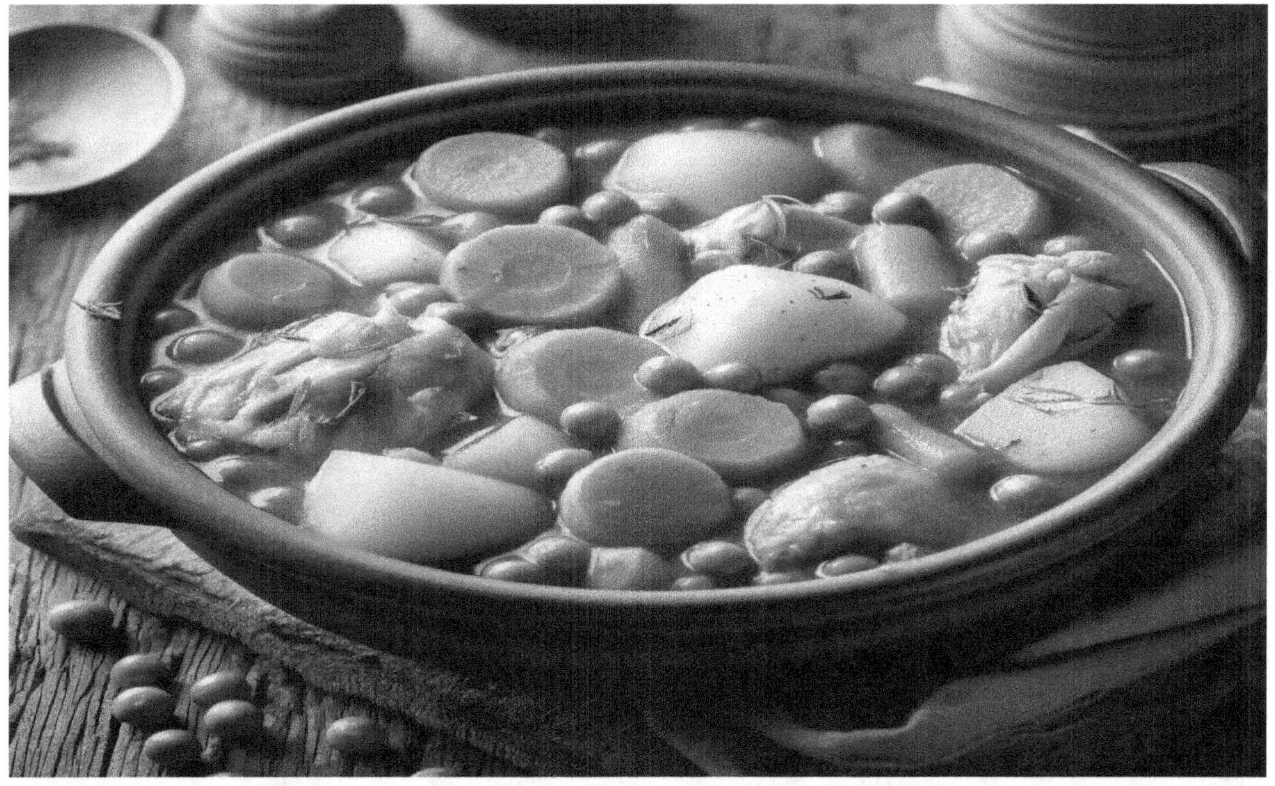

Chicken and Vegetable Stew

Nutritional Information: Calories: 240, Protein: 26g, Carbohydrates: 23g, Fat: 4g, Fiber: 5g, Sodium: 420mg.

Ingredients:

- 2 boneless, skinless chicken breasts, cubed
- 2 carrots, peeled and sliced
- 2 potatoes, peeled and cubed
- 1 cup peas
- 1 onion, chopped
- 3 cups chicken broth
- 1 teaspoon thyme
- Salt and pepper to taste

Prep Time: 10 minutes, **Cook Time**: 35 minutes, **Servings**: 4

Instructions:

1. In a large pot, heat a little oil over medium heat and sauté the onion until translucent.
2. Add chicken and brown on all sides.
3. Add carrots, potatoes, thyme, and chicken broth. Bring to a boil.
4. Reduce heat and simmer for 25 minutes.
5. Add peas and cook for another 10 minutes. Season with salt and pepper.

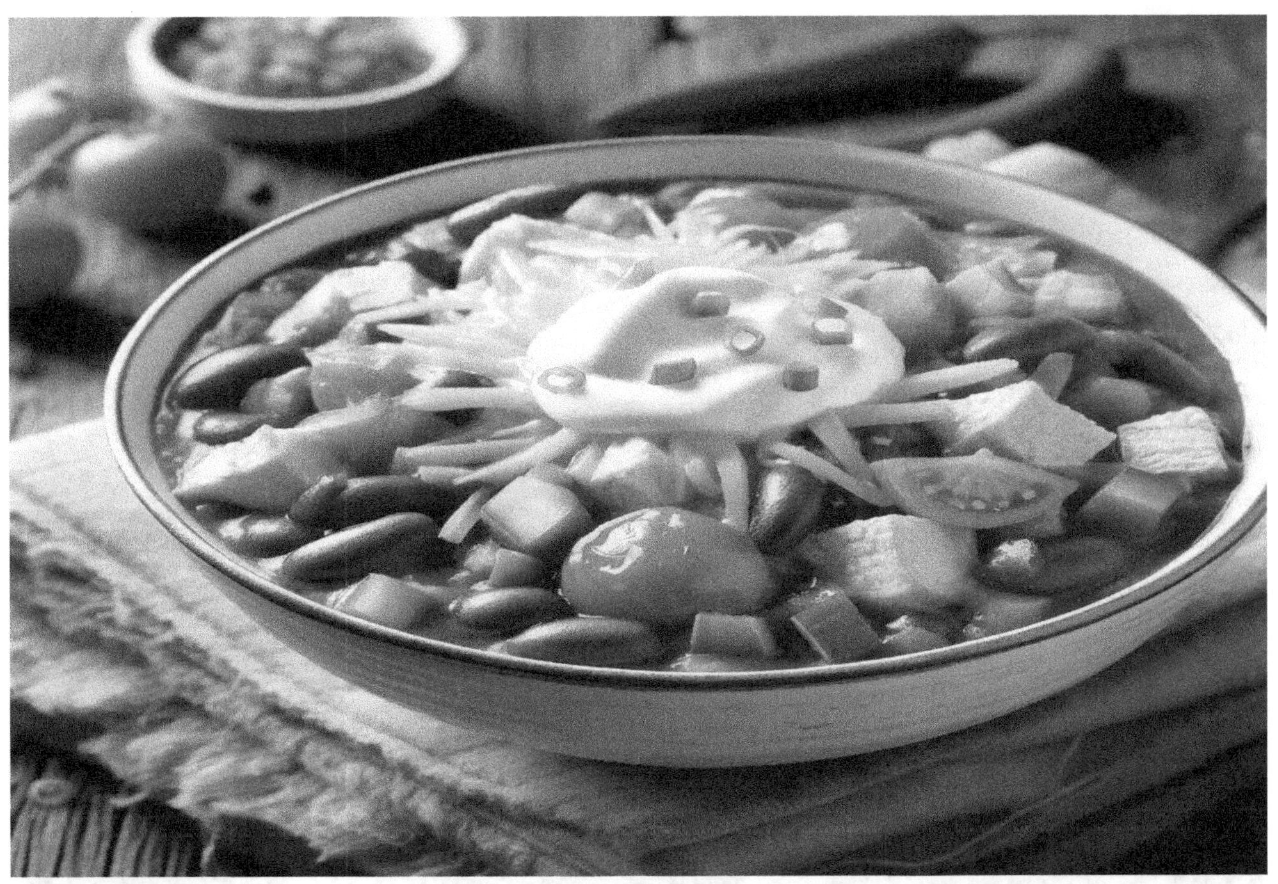

Nutritional Information: Calories: 330, Protein: 28g, Carbohydrates: 27g, Fat: 12g, Fiber: 6g, Sodium: 460mg.

Ingredients:

- 1 pound ground turkey
- 1 can kidney beans, drained and rinsed
- 2 cups tomato sauce
- 1 bell pepper, diced
- 1 onion, diced
- 2 garlic cloves, minced
- 1 tablespoon chili powder
- 1 teaspoon cumin
- Salt and pepper to taste
- Greek yogurt and cheddar cheese for topping

Prep Time: 15 minutes, **Cook Time**: 30 minutes, **Servings**: 4

Instructions:

1. In a pot, sauté onion, garlic, and bell pepper until soft.

2. Add ground turkey and cook until browned.

3. Stir in kidney beans, tomato sauce, chili powder, and cumin.

4. Simmer for 20 minutes. Season with salt and pepper.

5. Serve topped with a dollop of Greek yogurt and a sprinkle of cheddar cheese.

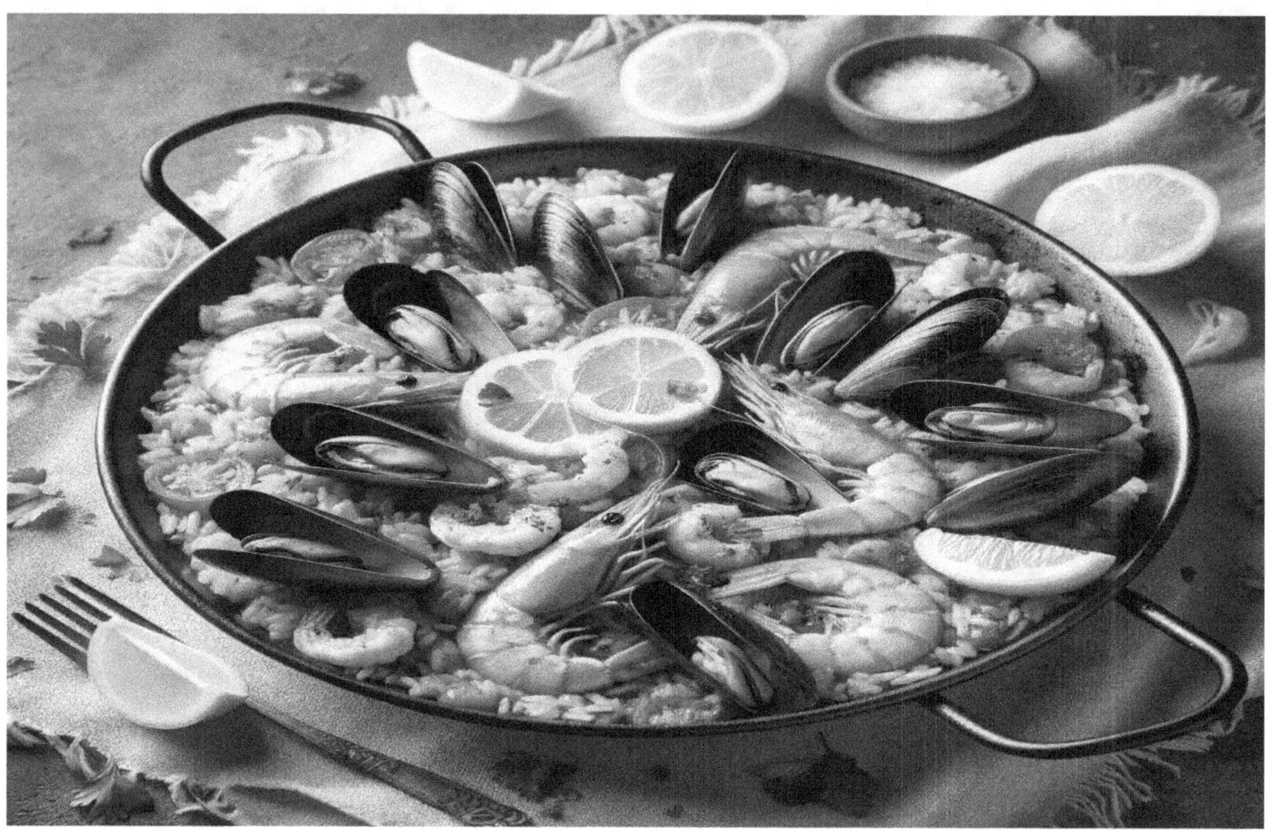

Seafood Paella

Nutritional Information: Calories: 320, Protein: 24g, Carbohydrates: 40g, Fat: 6g, Fiber: 3g, Sodium: 480mg.

Ingredients:

- 8 oz shrimp, peeled and deveined
- 4 oz mussels, cleaned
- 4 oz white fish, cubed
- 1 cup rice
- 3 cups fish broth
- 1/2 teaspoon saffron
- 1 bell pepper, sliced
- 1 onion, chopped
- 1 tomato, chopped
- Lemon slices and parsley for garnish

Prep Time: 15 minutes, **Cook Time**: 30 minutes, **Servings**: 4

Instructions:

1. In a large pan, sauté onion, bell pepper, and tomato until soft.

2. Add rice, saffron, and fish broth. Bring to a boil, then reduce to a simmer.

3. When rice is half-cooked, add shrimp, mussels, and white fish.

4. Cook until seafood is done and rice is tender.

5. Garnish with lemon slices and parsley before serving.

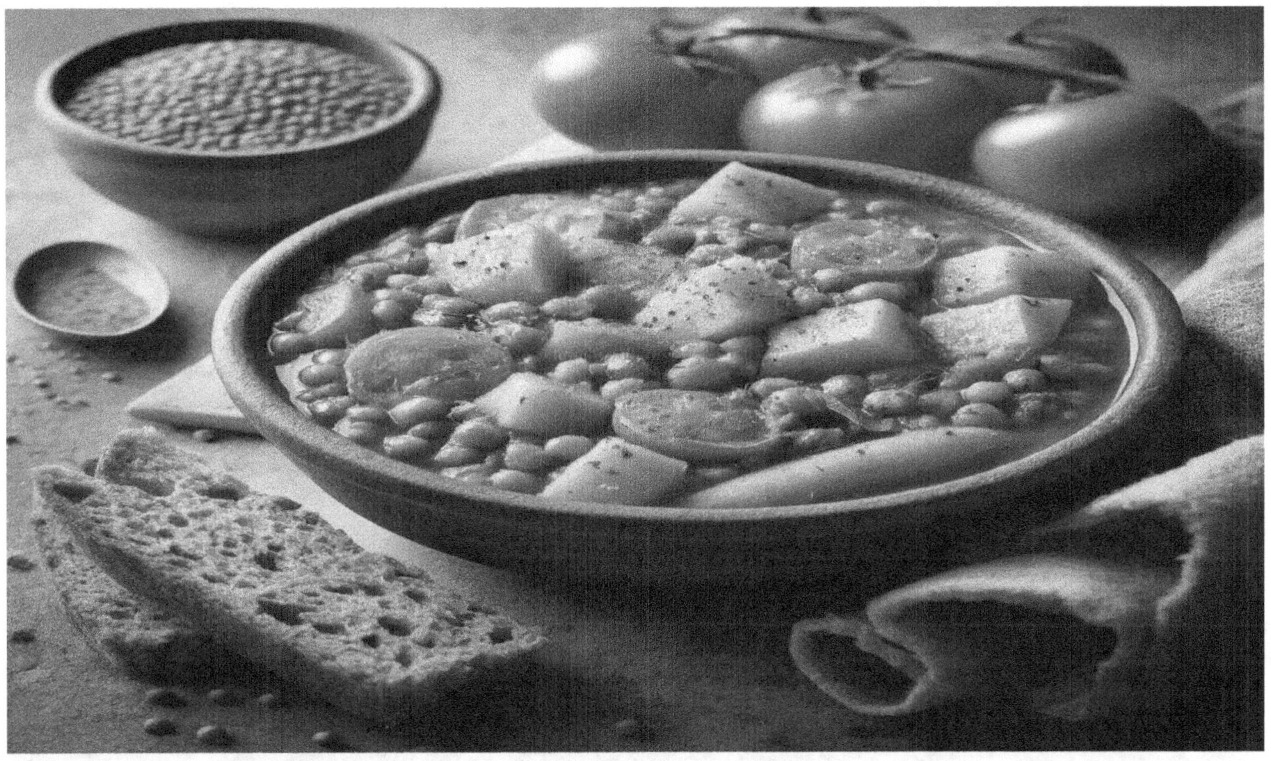

Lentil and Sweet Potato Stew

Nutritional Information: Calories: 260, Protein: 12g, Carbohydrates: 45g, Fat: 2g, Fiber: 9g, Sodium: 300mg.

Ingredients:

- 1 cup lentils, rinsed
- 1 large sweet potato, cubed
- 2 carrots, sliced
- 1 onion, chopped
- 3 cups vegetable broth
- 1 teaspoon cumin
- 1 teaspoon coriander
- Salt and pepper to taste

Prep Time: 10 minutes, **Cook Time**: 25 minutes, **Servings**: 4

Instructions:

1. In a large pot, sauté onion until translucent.

2. Add sweet potatoes, carrots, lentils, cumin, and coriander. Stir to combine.

3. Pour in vegetable broth and bring to a boil.

4. Reduce heat and simmer until lentils and vegetables are tender, about 20 minutes.

5. Season with salt and pepper.

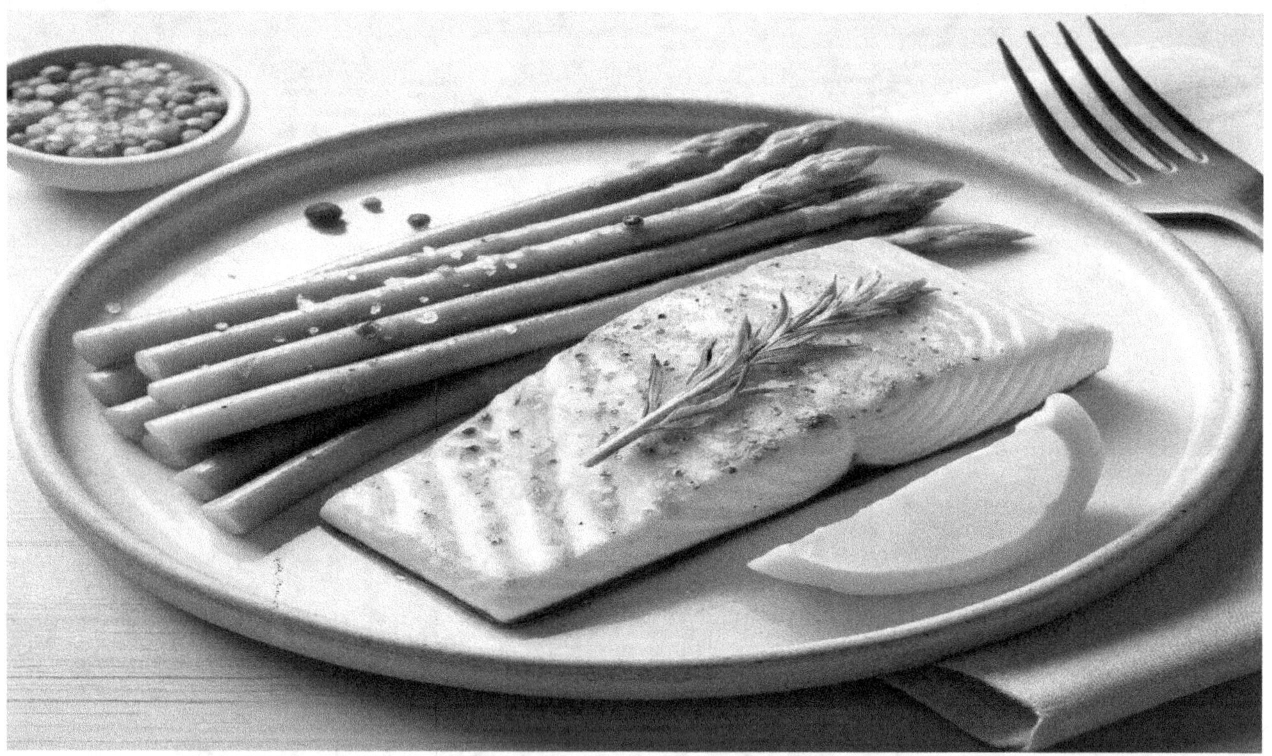

Grilled Salmon with Steamed Asparagus

Nutritional Information: Calories: 345, Protein: 34g, Carbohydrates: 5g, Fat: 20g, Fiber: 2g, Sodium: 75mg.

Ingredients:

- 1 salmon fillet (about 6 oz)
- 1 cup asparagus spears
- 1 tablespoon olive oil
- 1 lemon wedge
- Salt and pepper to taste

Prep Time: 5 minutes, **Cook Time**: 10 minutes, **Servings**: 1

Instructions:

1. Preheat grill or pan to medium-high heat.

2. Brush salmon and asparagus with olive oil; season with salt and pepper.

3. Grill salmon for about 5 minutes per side or until cooked through.

4. Steam asparagus until tender, about 3-5 minutes.

5. Serve salmon and asparagus with a squeeze of lemon.

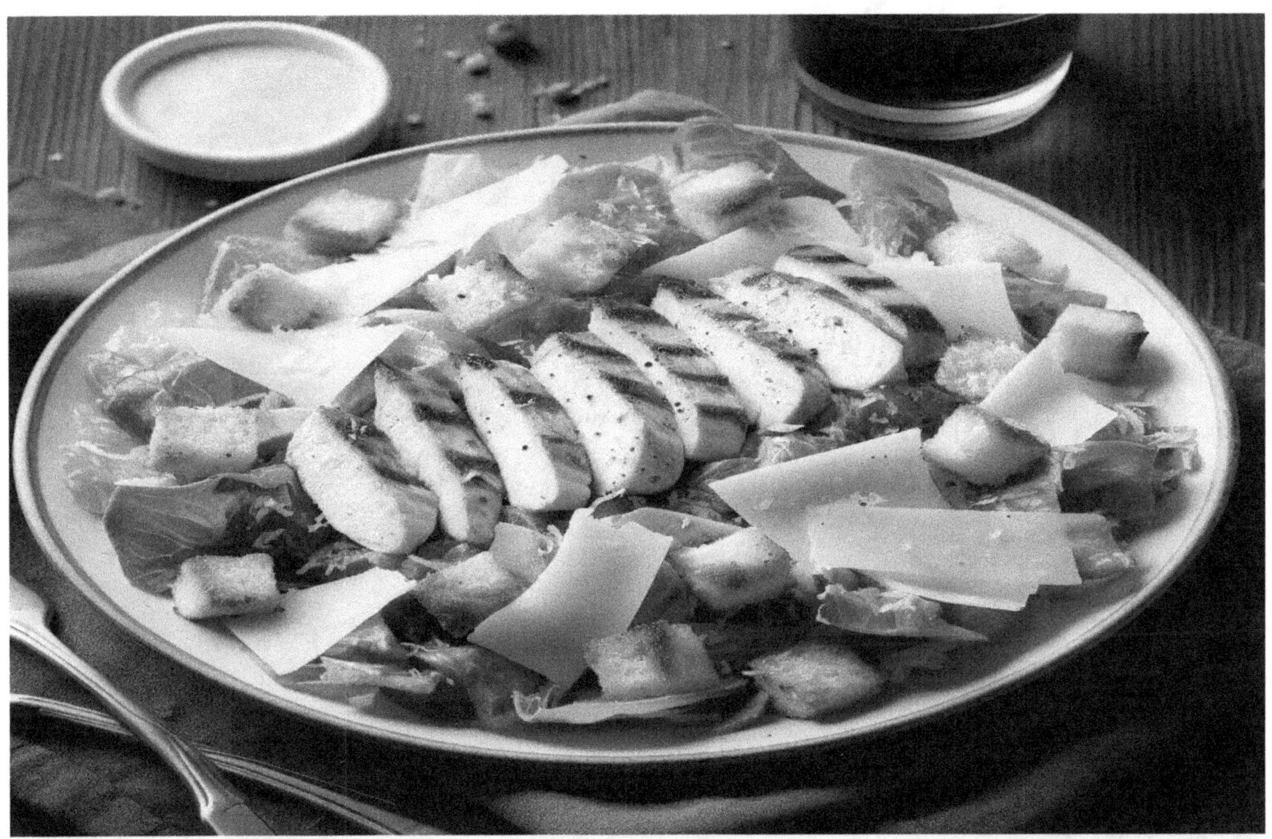

Light Chicken Caesar Salad

Nutritional Information: Calories: 290, Protein: 28g, Carbohydrates: 14g, Fat: 12g, Fiber: 2g, Sodium: 420mg.

Ingredients:

- 1 chicken breast, grilled and sliced
- 2 cups romaine lettuce, chopped
- 1/4 cup croutons

- 2 tablespoons low-fat Caesar dressing
- 1 tablespoon Parmesan cheese, shaved
- Salt and pepper to taste

Prep Time: 10 minutes, **Cook Time**: 10 minutes, **Servings**: 1

Instructions:

1. Toss romaine lettuce with Caesar dressing in a bowl.
2. Top with grilled chicken, croutons, and Parmesan cheese.
3. Season with salt and pepper to taste.

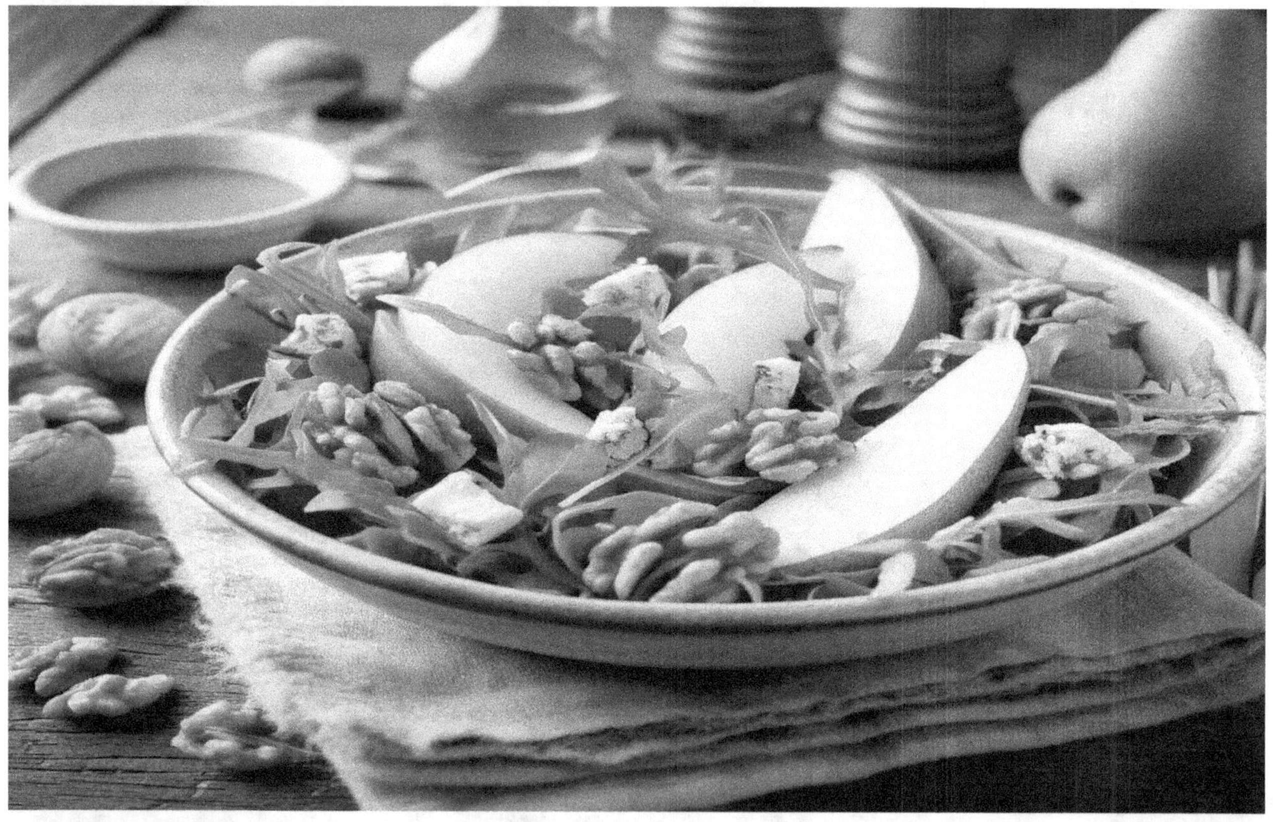

Arugula and Pear Salad with Blue Cheese

Nutritional Information: Calories: 275, Protein: 7g, Carbohydrates: 22g, Fat: 18g, Fiber: 5g, Sodium: 320mg.

Ingredients:

- 2 cups arugula
- 1 pear, thinly sliced
- 1/4 cup crumbled blue cheese
- 1/4 cup walnuts, chopped

- 2 tablespoons balsamic vinaigrette

Prep Time: 5 minutes, **Cook Time**: 0 minutes, **Servings**: 1

Instructions:

1. Combine arugula, pear slices, and walnuts in a salad bowl.

2. Drizzle with balsamic vinaigrette and toss to coat.

3. Top with crumbled blue cheese.

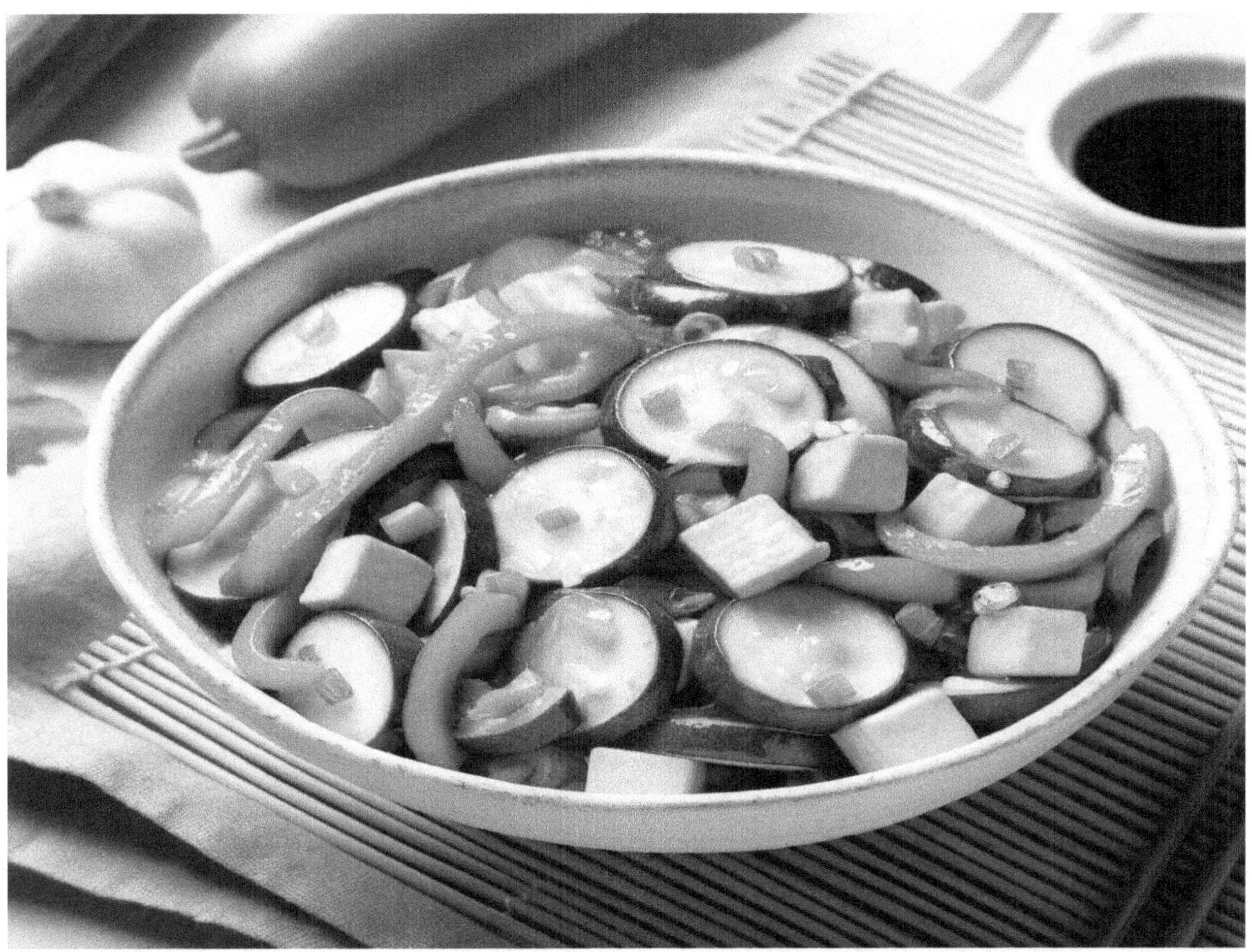

Vegetable Tofu Stir-Fry

Nutritional Information: Calories: 225, Protein: 12g, Carbohydrates: 10g, Fat: 15g, Fiber: 3g, Sodium: 330mg.

Ingredients:

- 1/2 block firm tofu, cubed

- 1/2 zucchini, sliced

- 1/2 bell pepper, sliced
- 1 tablespoon soy sauce
- 1 teaspoon sesame oil
- 1 garlic clove, minced

Prep Time: 10 minutes, **Cook Time**: 10 minutes, **Servings**: 1

Instructions:

1. Heat sesame oil in a skillet over medium heat.

2. Add tofu and vegetables, stir-frying until golden and tender.

3. Add garlic and soy sauce, stir-fry for another 2 minutes.

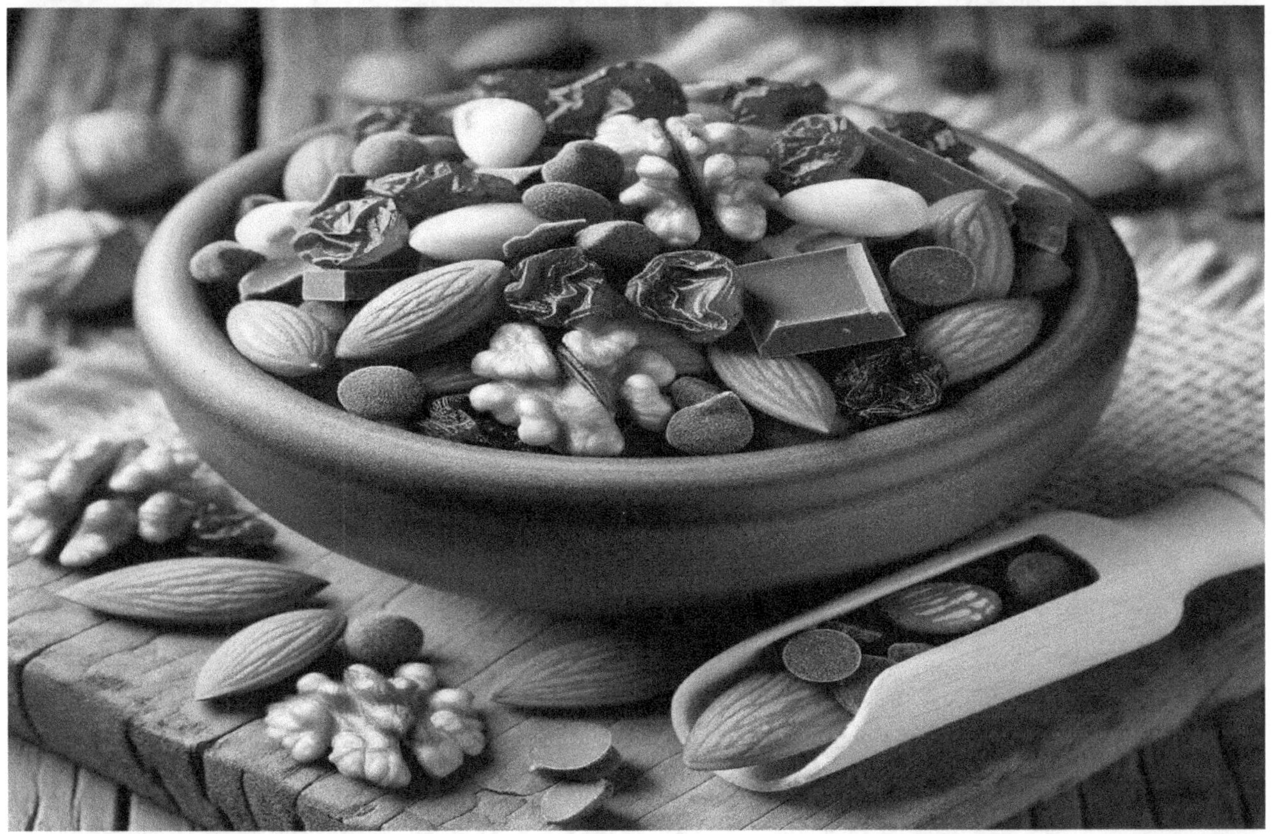

Homemade Trail Mix

Nutritional Information: Calories: 200, Protein: 4g, Carbohydrates: 15g, Fat: 14g, Fiber: 3g, Sodium: 10mg.

Ingredients:

- 1/4 cup almonds
- 1/4 cup walnuts
- 1/4 cup dried cranberries
- 2 tablespoons dark chocolate chips

Prep Time: 5 minutes, **Cook Time**: 0 minutes, **Servings**: 4

Instructions:

1. Combine all ingredients in a bowl and mix well.

2. Divide into portions and store in small bags or containers for easy snacking.

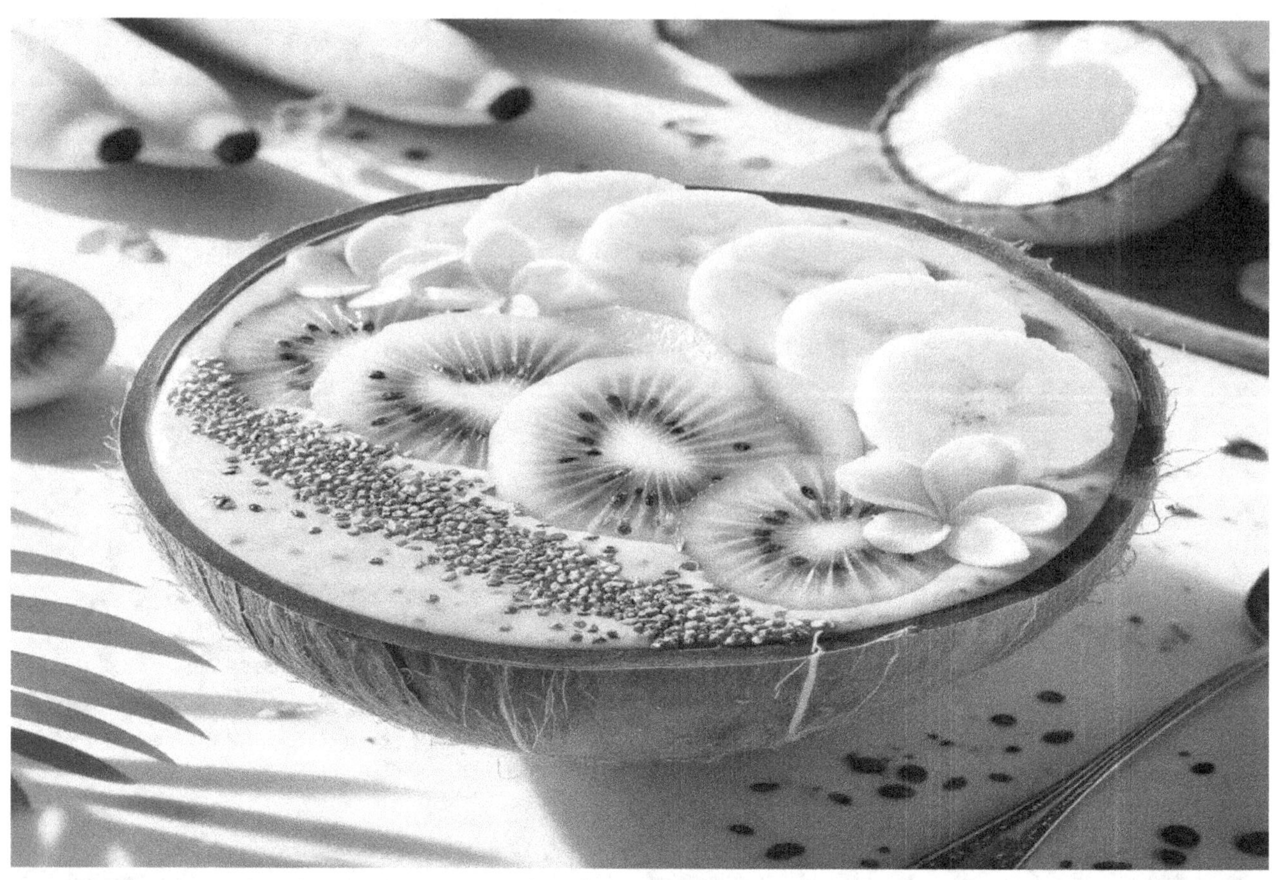

Banana Kiwi Smoothie Bowl

Nutritional Information: Calories: 285, Protein: 5g, Carbohydrates: 53g, Fat: 7g, Fiber: 9g, Sodium: 30mg.

Ingredients:

- 1 banana
- 1 kiwi, peeled and sliced
- 1/2 cup almond milk
- 1 tablespoon chia seeds

Prep Time: 10 minutes, **Blend Time**: 2 minutes, Servings: 1

Instructions:

1. Blend the banana and almond milk until smooth.

2. Pour into a bowl and top with kiwi slices and chia seeds.

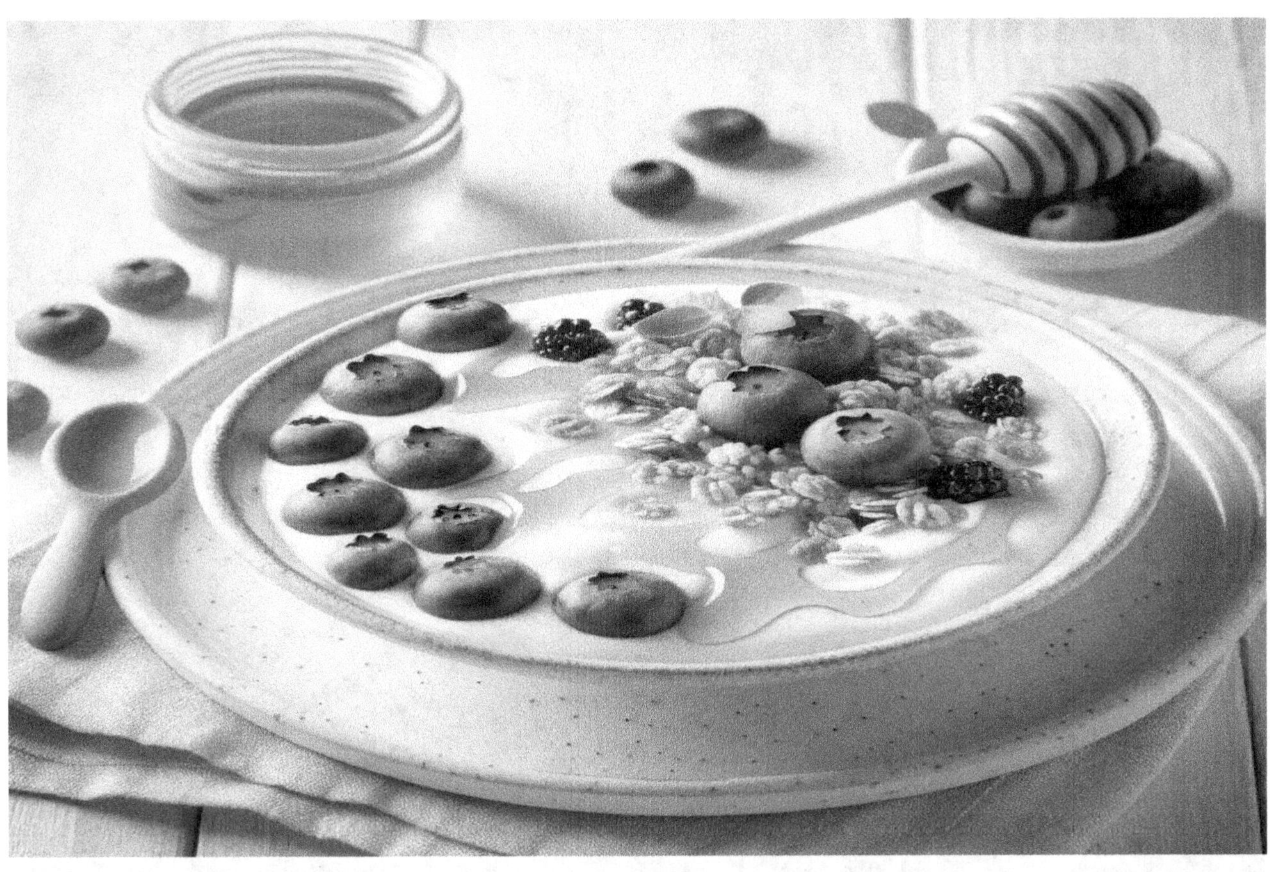

Greek Yogurt with Granola and Blueberries

Nutritional Information: Calories: 290, Protein: 20g, Carbohydrates: 35g, Fat: 9g, Fiber: 3g, Sodium: 70mg.

Ingredients:

- 1 cup Greek yogurt, low-fat
- 1/4 cup granola
- 1/4 cup fresh blueberries
- 1 tablespoon honey

Prep Time: 5 minutes, **Cook Time**: 0 minutes, **Servings**: 1

Instructions:

1. Spoon Greek yogurt into a bowl.
2. Top with granola, blueberries, and drizzle with honey.

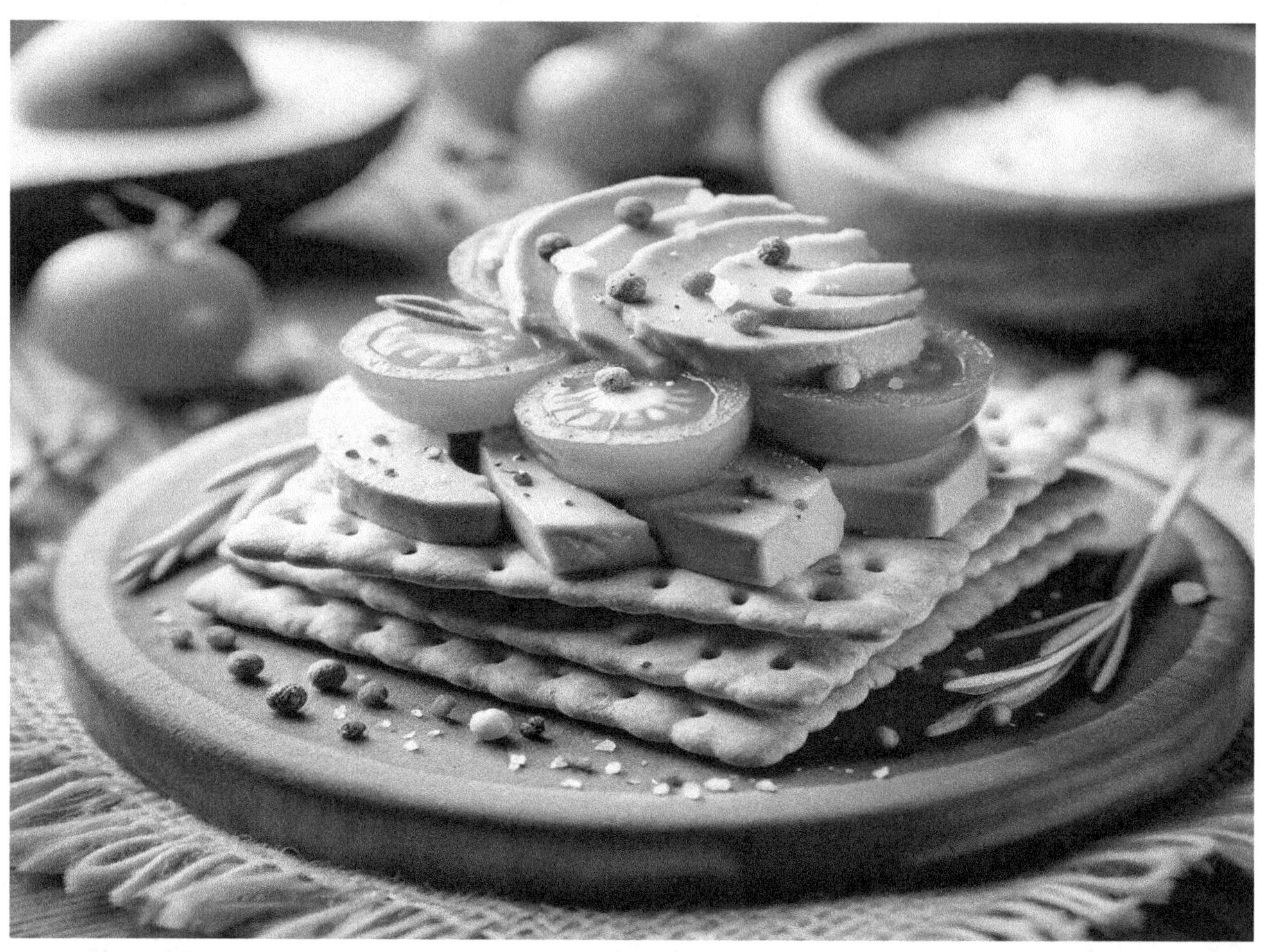

Avocado and Tomato Crackers

Nutritional Information: Calories: 250, Protein: 5g, Carbohydrates: 20g, Fat: 18g, Fiber: 7g, Sodium: 150mg.

Ingredients:

- 4 whole grain crackers
- 1/2 avocado, sliced
- 4 cherry tomatoes, halved
- Sea salt and black pepper to taste

Prep Time: 5 minutes, **Cook Time**: 0 minutes, **Servings**: 1

Instructions:

1. Top each cracker with slices of avocado and two halves of cherry tomato.
2. Sprinkle with sea salt and black pepper.

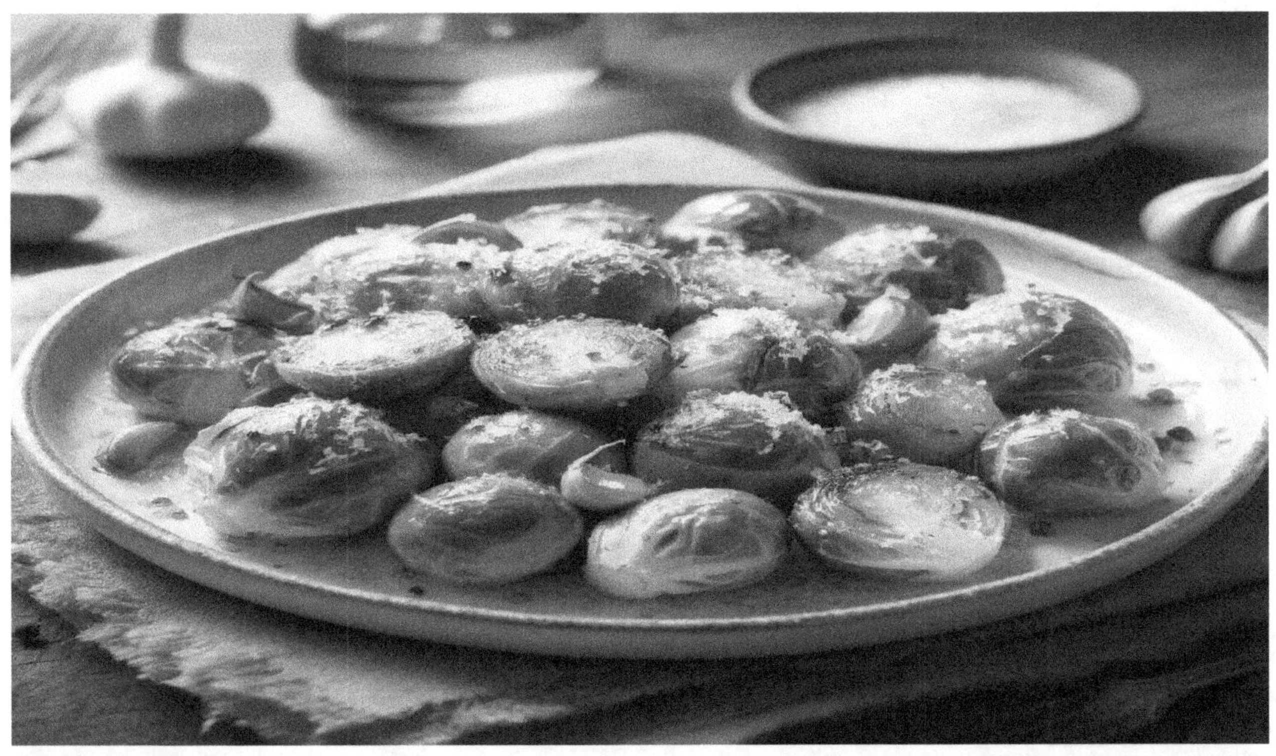

Roasted Brussels Sprouts with Garlic

Nutritional Information: Calories: 120, Protein: 5g, Carbohydrates: 10g, Fat: 7g, Fiber: 4g, Sodium: 55mg.

Ingredients:

- 1 lb Brussels sprouts, halved
- 2 tablespoons olive oil
- 2 cloves garlic, minced
- Salt and pepper to taste
- 2 tablespoons grated Parmesan cheese

Prep Time: 5 minutes, **Cook Time**: 20 minutes, **Servings**: 4

Instructions:

1. Preheat oven to 400°F (200°C).
2. Toss Brussels sprouts with olive oil, garlic, salt, and pepper.
3. Spread on a baking sheet and roast for 20 minutes, until crisp on the outside and tender inside.
4. Sprinkle with Parmesan cheese before serving.

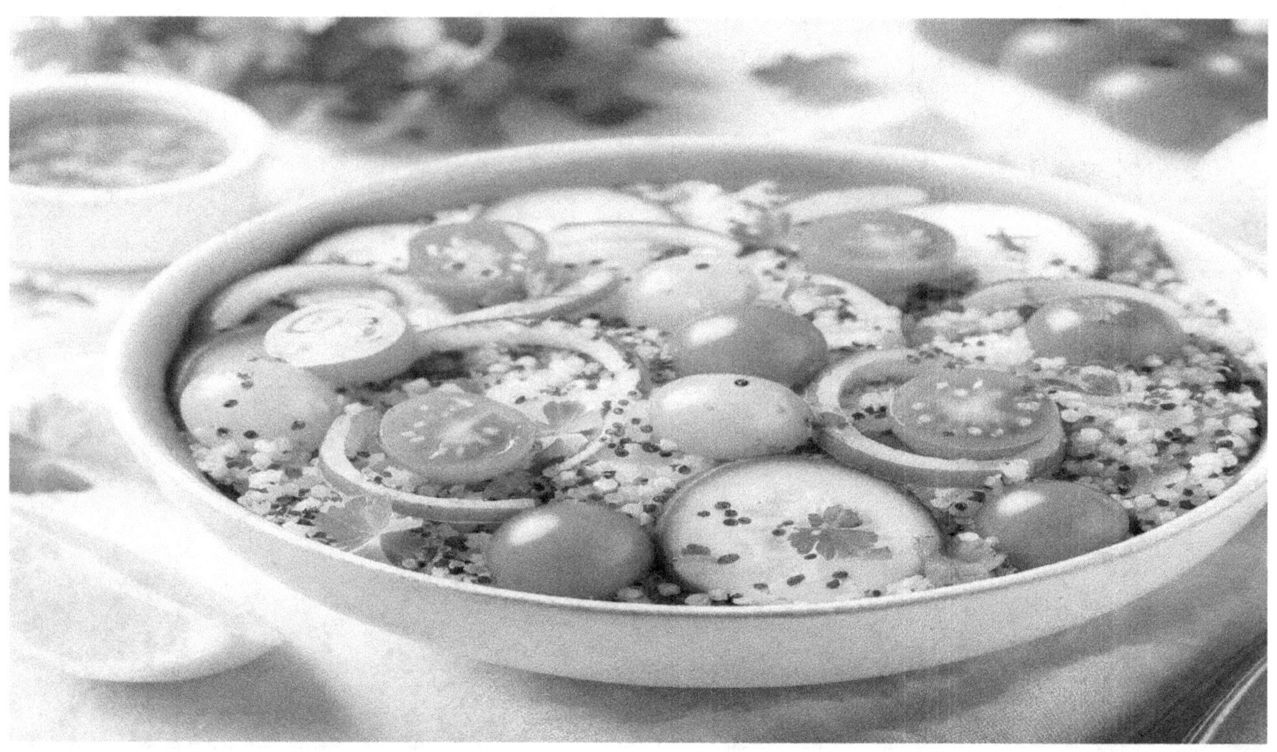

Quinoa Salad with Vegetables

Nutritional Information: Calories: 250, Protein: 6g, Carbohydrates: 30g, Fat: 12g, Fiber: 4g, Sodium: 30mg

Ingredients:

- 1 cup quinoa
- 2 cups water
- 1/2 cup cherry tomatoes, halved
- 1/2 cucumber, diced
- 1/4 red onion, finely chopped
- 1/4 cup fresh parsley, chopped
- 2 tablespoons lemon juice
- 3 tablespoons olive oil
- Salt and pepper to taste

Prep Time: 10 minutes, **Cook Time**: 15 minutes, **Servings**: 4

Instructions:

1. Rinse quinoa under cold water. In a pot, bring quinoa and water to a boil. Reduce heat to low, cover, and simmer for 15 minutes.
2. Fluff quinoa with a fork and let it cool.
3. Add tomatoes, cucumber, onion, and parsley to the quinoa.

4. Whisk together lemon juice, olive oil, salt, and pepper. Pour over the salad and mix well.

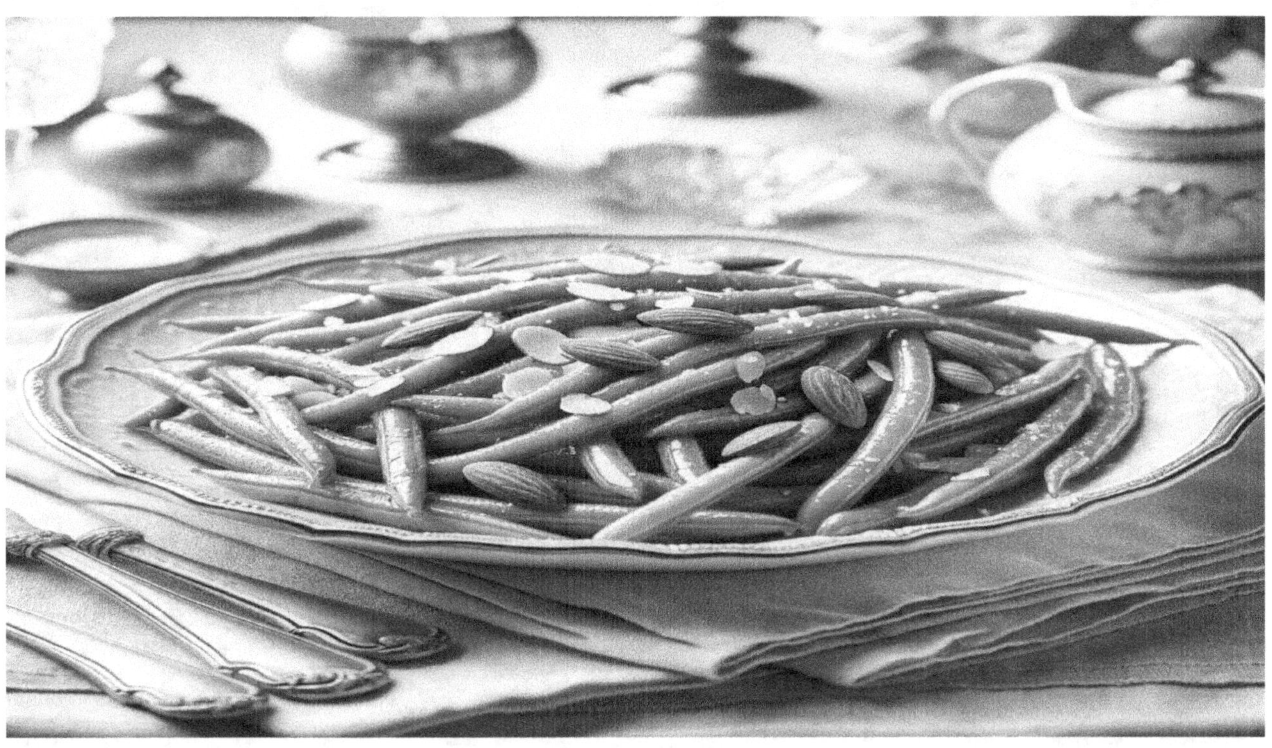

Steamed Green Beans with Almonds

Nutritional Information: Calories: 100, Protein: 3g, Carbohydrates: 8g, Fat: 7g, Fiber: 3g, Sodium: 55mg.

Ingredients:

- 1 lb green beans, ends trimmed
- 1/4 cup slivered almonds
- 1 tablespoon butter
- Salt and pepper to taste

Prep Time: 5 minutes, **Cook Time**: 10 minutes, **Servings**: 4

Instructions:

1. Steam green beans until tender, about 7-10 minutes.

2. In a skillet, toast almonds over medium heat until golden.

3. Toss steamed green beans with butter, toasted almonds, salt, and pepper.

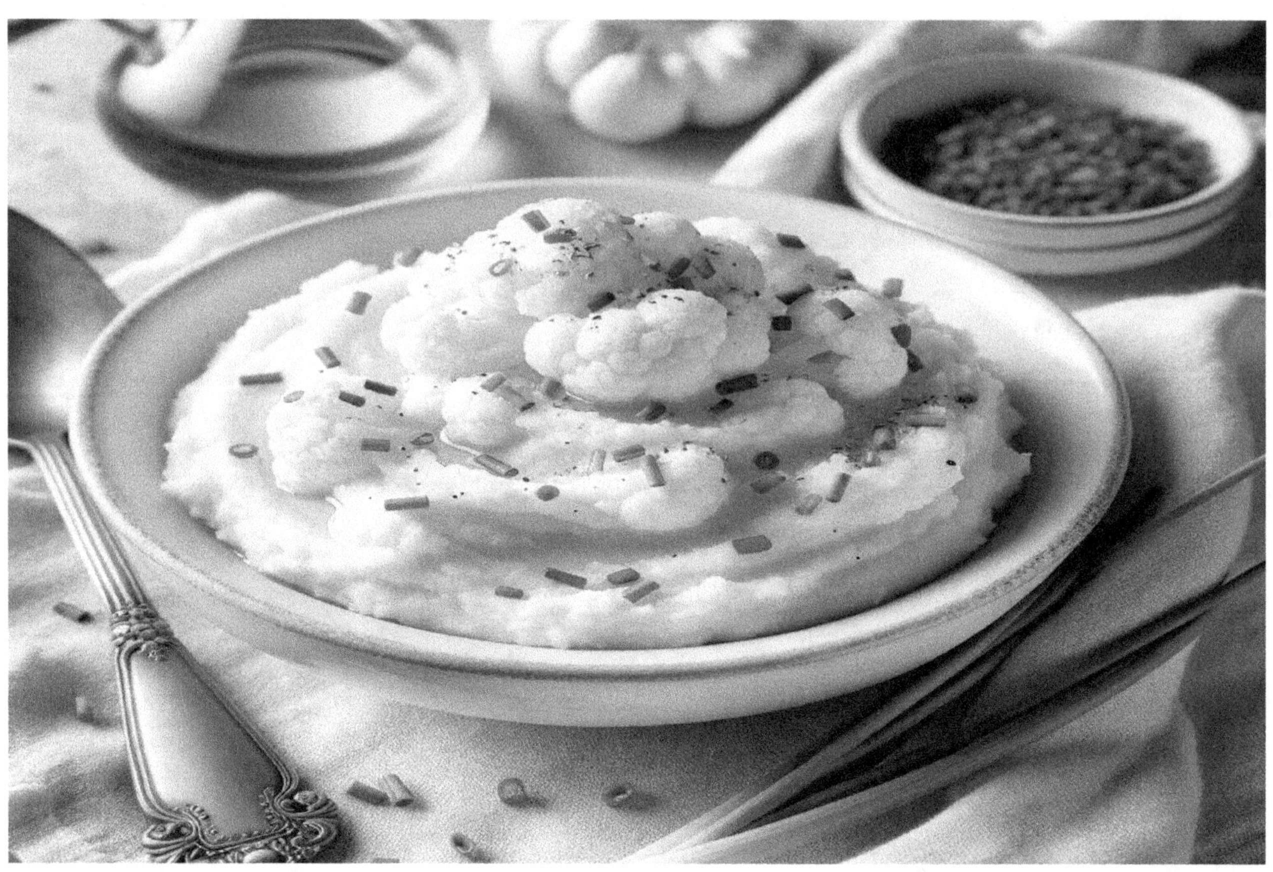

Mashed Cauliflower with Chives

Nutritional Information: Calories: 120, Protein: 2g, Carbohydrates: 10g, Fat: 9g, Fiber: 4g, Sodium: 30mg.

Ingredients:

- 1 head cauliflower, cut into florets
- 2 tablespoons olive oil
- 1/4 cup fresh chives, chopped
- Salt and pepper to taste

Prep Time: 10 minutes, **Cook Time**: 15 minutes, **Servings**: 4

Instructions:

1. Steam cauliflower florets until very tender, about 15 minutes.
2. Mash cauliflower with olive oil until smooth.
3. Stir in chives, salt, and pepper.

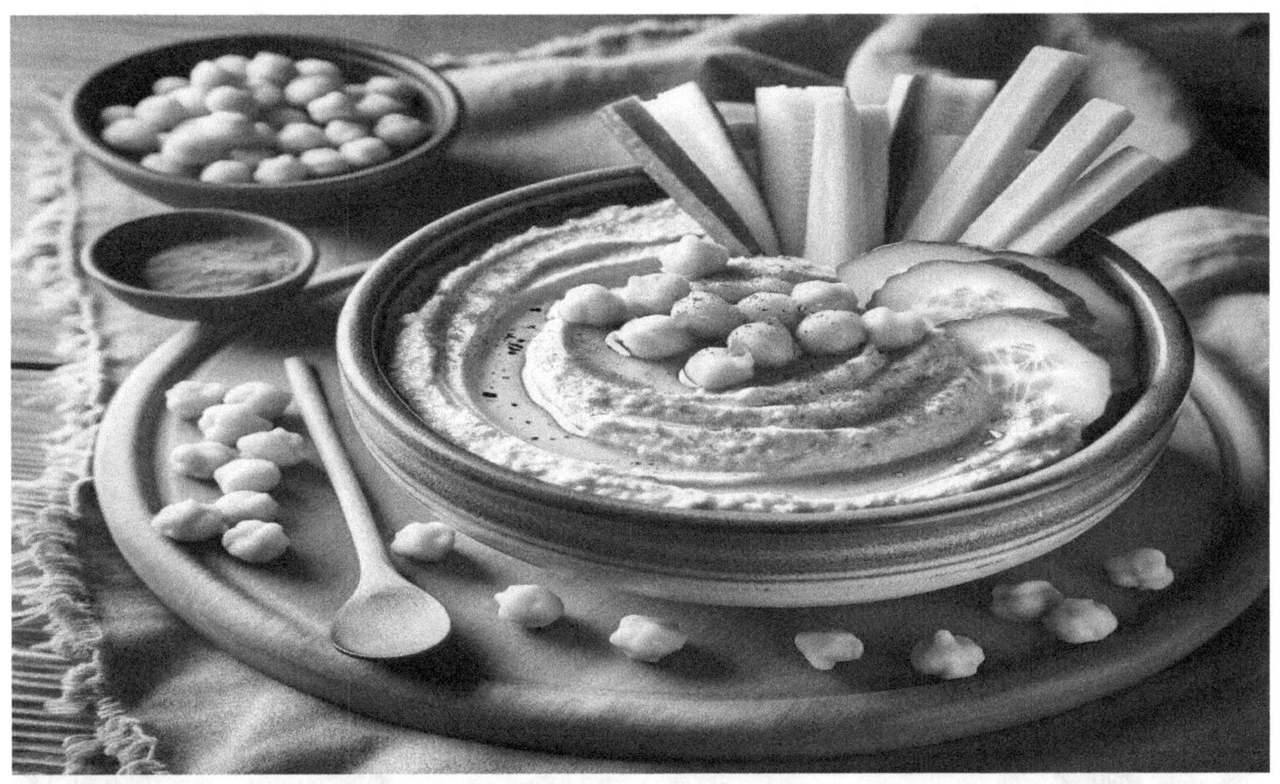

Creamy Avocado Hummus

Nutritional Information: Calories: 200, Protein: 6g, Carbohydrates: 20g, Fat: 12g, Fiber: 6g, Sodium: 200mg.

Ingredients:

- 1 ripe avocado
- 1 can (15 oz) chickpeas, drained and rinsed
- 2 tablespoons olive oil
- 1 clove garlic, minced
- Juice of 1 lemon
- Salt and paprika to taste

Prep Time: 10 minutes, **Cook Time**: 0 minutes, **Servings**: 4

Instructions:

1. In a food processor, combine all ingredients except for paprika.
2. Blend until smooth and creamy.
3. Transfer to a serving bowl and sprinkle with paprika for garnish.
4. Serve with carrot sticks and cucumber slices.

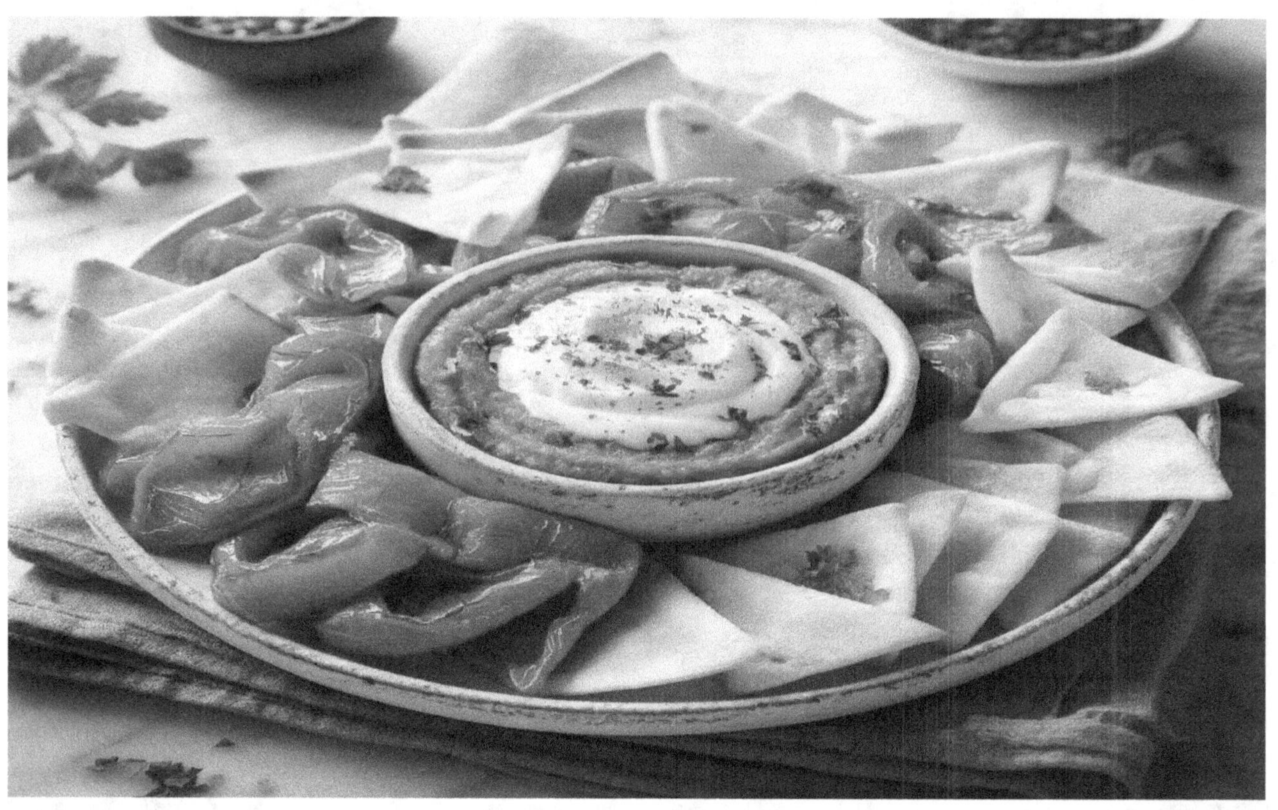

Roasted Red Pepper Dip

Nutritional Information: Calories: 90, Protein: 5g, Carbohydrates: 8g, Fat: 4.5g, Fiber: 1g, Sodium: 250mg.

Ingredients:

- 1 jar (12 oz) roasted red peppers, drained
- 1 cup Greek yogurt
- 1 clove garlic, minced
- 1 tablespoon olive oil
- Salt and pepper to taste
- Chopped parsley for garnish

Prep Time: 5 minutes, **Cook Time**: 0 minutes, **Servings**: 4

Instructions:

1. In a blender, combine roasted red peppers, Greek yogurt, garlic, and olive oil.
2. Blend until smooth.
3. Season with salt and pepper.
4. Garnish with parsley and serve with baked pita chips.

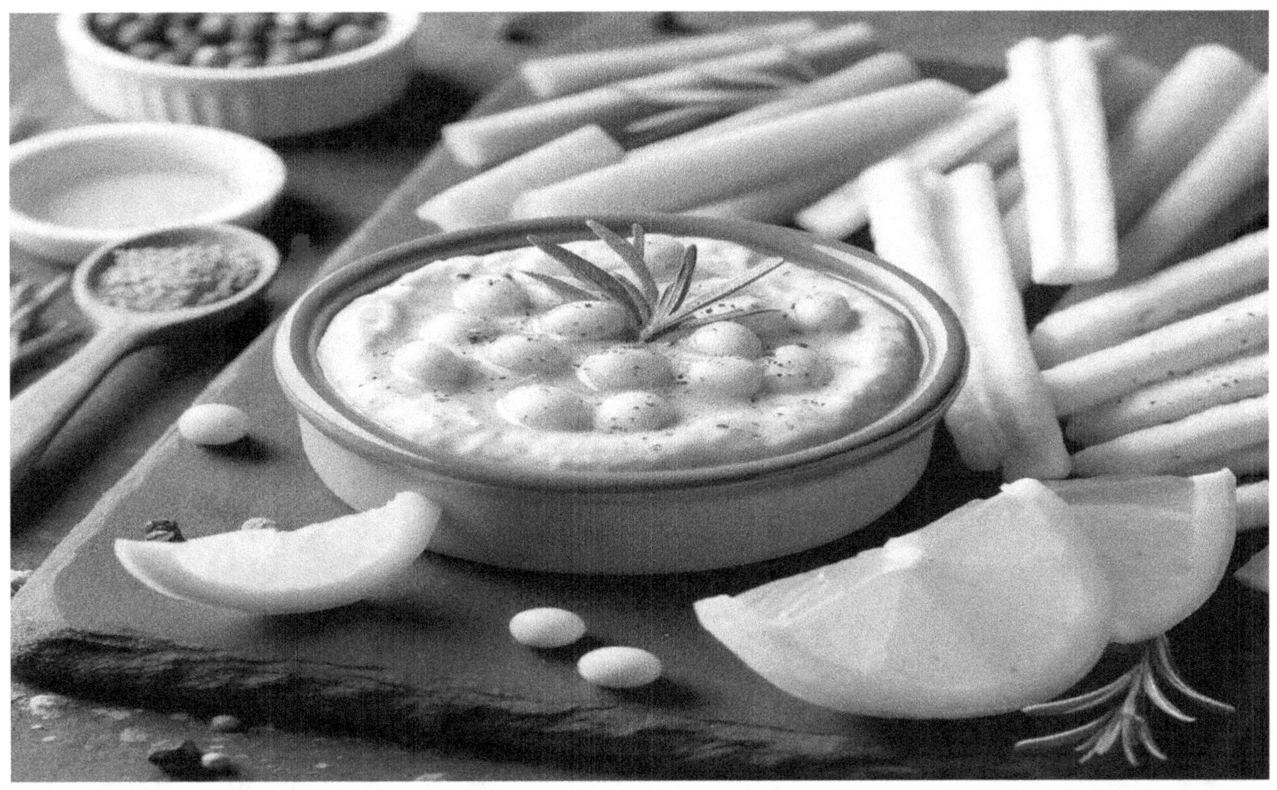

White Bean and Rosemary Dip

Nutritional Information: Calories: 150, Protein: 6g, Carbohydrates: 20g, Fat: 5g, Fiber: 5g, Sodium: 200mg.

Ingredients:

- 1 can (15 oz) white beans, drained and rinsed
- 2 tablespoons olive oil
- Juice of 1 lemon
- 1 teaspoon fresh rosemary, chopped
- Salt and cracked black pepper to taste

Prep Time: 5 minutes, **Cook Time**: 0 minutes, **Servings**: 4

Instructions:

1. In a food processor, combine white beans, olive oil, lemon juice, and rosemary.
2. Blend until smooth.
3. Season with salt and pepper.
4. Serve with vegetable sticks.

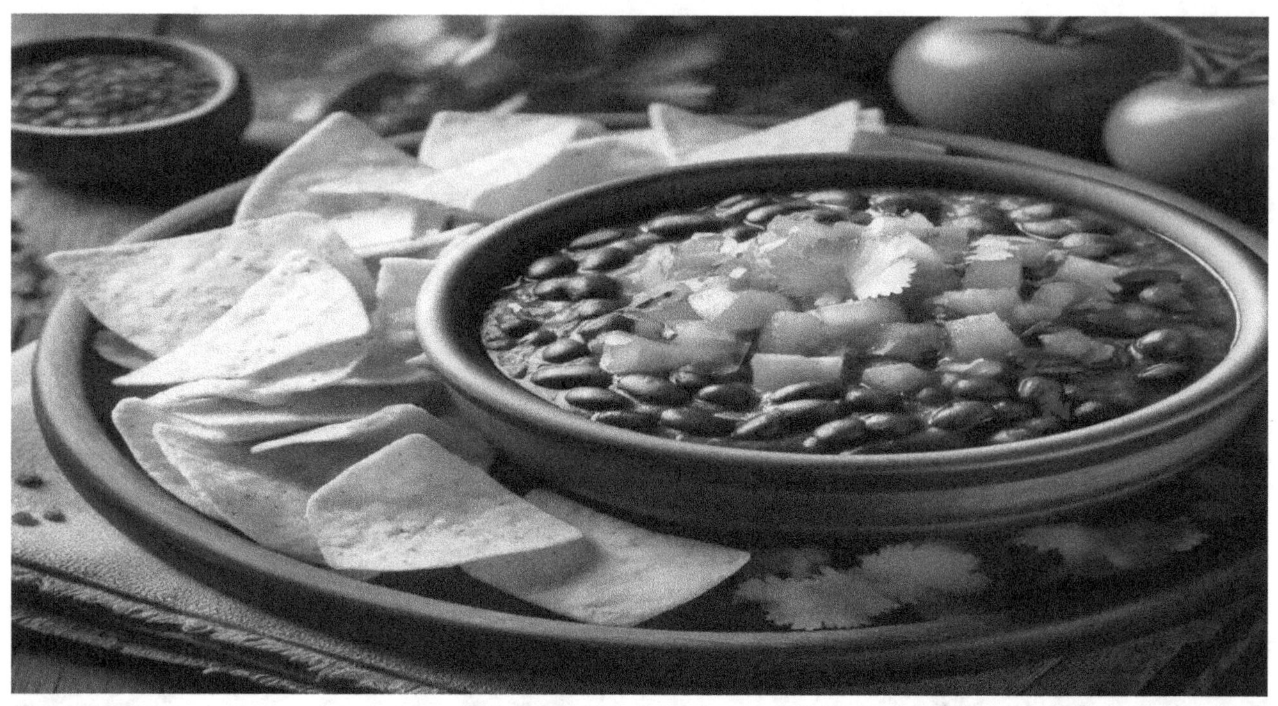

Spicy Black Bean Dip

Nutritional Information: Calories: 120, Protein: 7g, Carbohydrates: 20g, Fat: 2g, Fiber: 6g, Sodium: 200mg.

Ingredients:

- 1 can (15 oz) black beans, drained and rinsed
- 1 small tomato, diced
- 1/2 teaspoon cumin
- 1/2 teaspoon chili powder
- Juice of 1 lime
- Salt to taste
- Fresh cilantro, chopped for garnish

Prep Time: 10 minutes, **Cook Time**: 0 minutes, **Servings**: 4

Instructions:

1. In a food processor, blend black beans, cumin, chili powder, and lime juice until smooth.
2. Stir in diced tomatoes.
3. Season with salt.
4. Garnish with cilantro and serve with homemade corn tortilla chips.

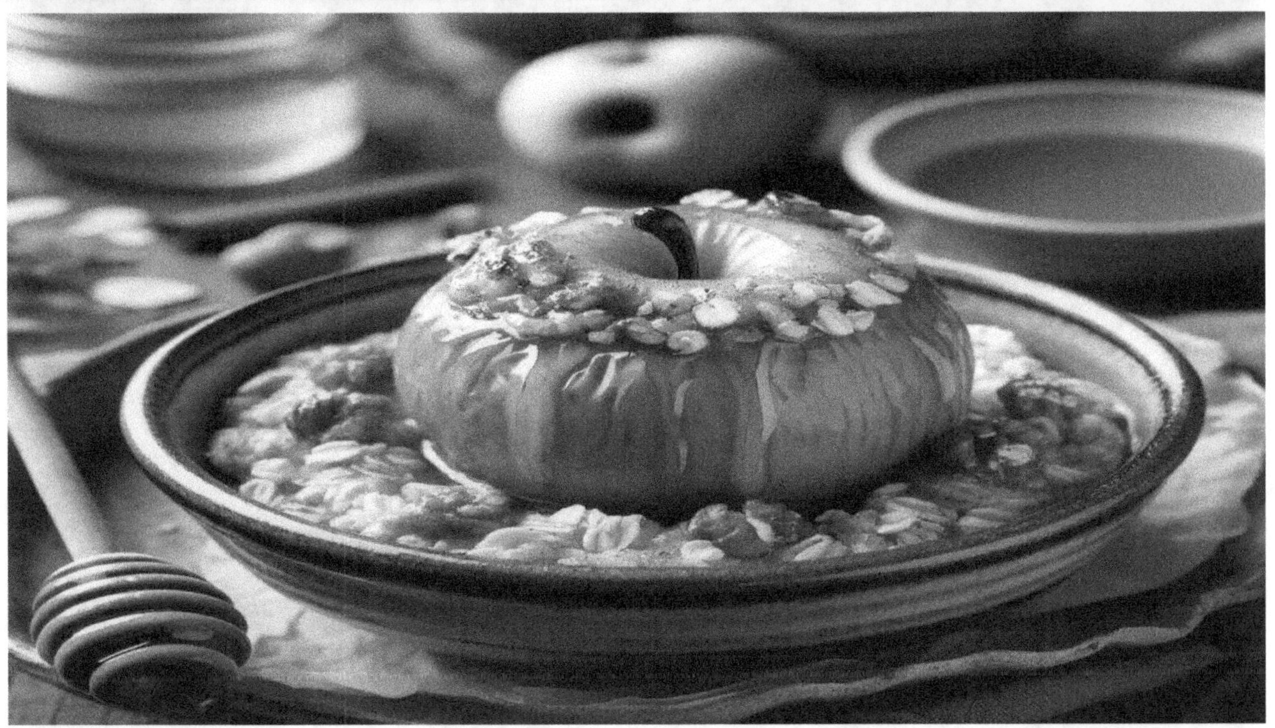

Baked Apples Stuffed with Oats and Nuts

Nutritional Information: Calories: 190, Protein: 2g, Carbohydrates: 35g, Fat: 4g, Fiber: 5g, Sodium: 5mg.

Ingredients:

- 4 large apples, cored
- 1/2 cup rolled oats
- 1/4 cup mixed nuts, chopped
- 1/4 cup dried cranberries
- 1/2 teaspoon cinnamon
- 2 tablespoons honey
- 1/2 cup water

Prep Time: 10 minutes, **Cook Time**: 30 minutes, **Servings**: 4

Instructions:

1. Preheat oven to 350°F (175°C).
2. Mix oats, nuts, cranberries, cinnamon, and 1 tablespoon honey in a bowl.
3. Stuff each apple with the oat mixture and place in a baking dish.

4. Drizzle remaining honey over the apples and add water to the dish.

5. Bake for 30 minutes or until apples are tender.

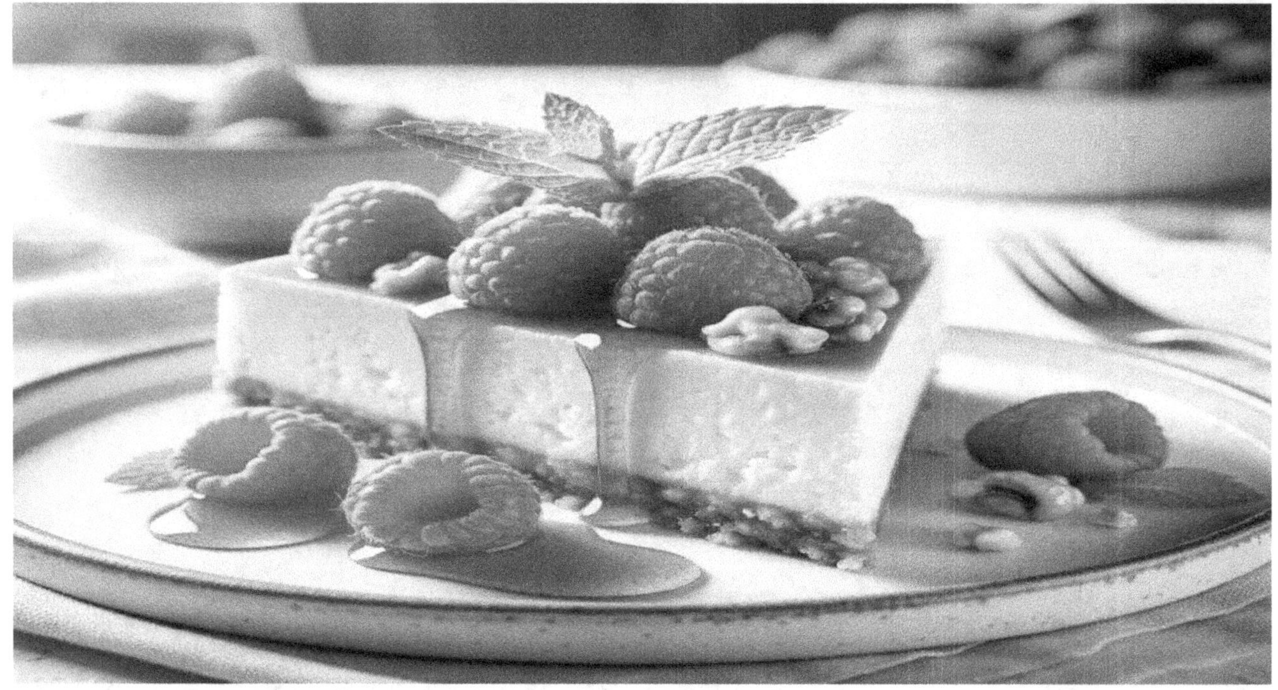

No-Bake Cheesecake with Raspberries

Nutritional Information: Calories: 250, Protein: 6g, Carbohydrates: 28g, Fat: 14g, Fiber: 4g, Sodium: 20mg.

Ingredients:

- 1 cup crushed nuts (almonds, walnuts)
- 1 cup Greek yogurt, low-fat
- 1/4 cup agave syrup
- 1 teaspoon vanilla extract
- 1/2 cup fresh raspberries
- Mint leaves for garnish

Prep Time: 15 minutes, **Chill Time**: 2 hours, **Servings**: 4

Instructions:

1. Mix crushed nuts and 2 tablespoons agave syrup to form the crust. Press into the bottom of a serving dish.

2. Blend Greek yogurt, remaining agave syrup, and vanilla until smooth.

3. Pour over the nut crust and refrigerate for at least 2 hours.

4. Top with fresh raspberries and mint before serving.

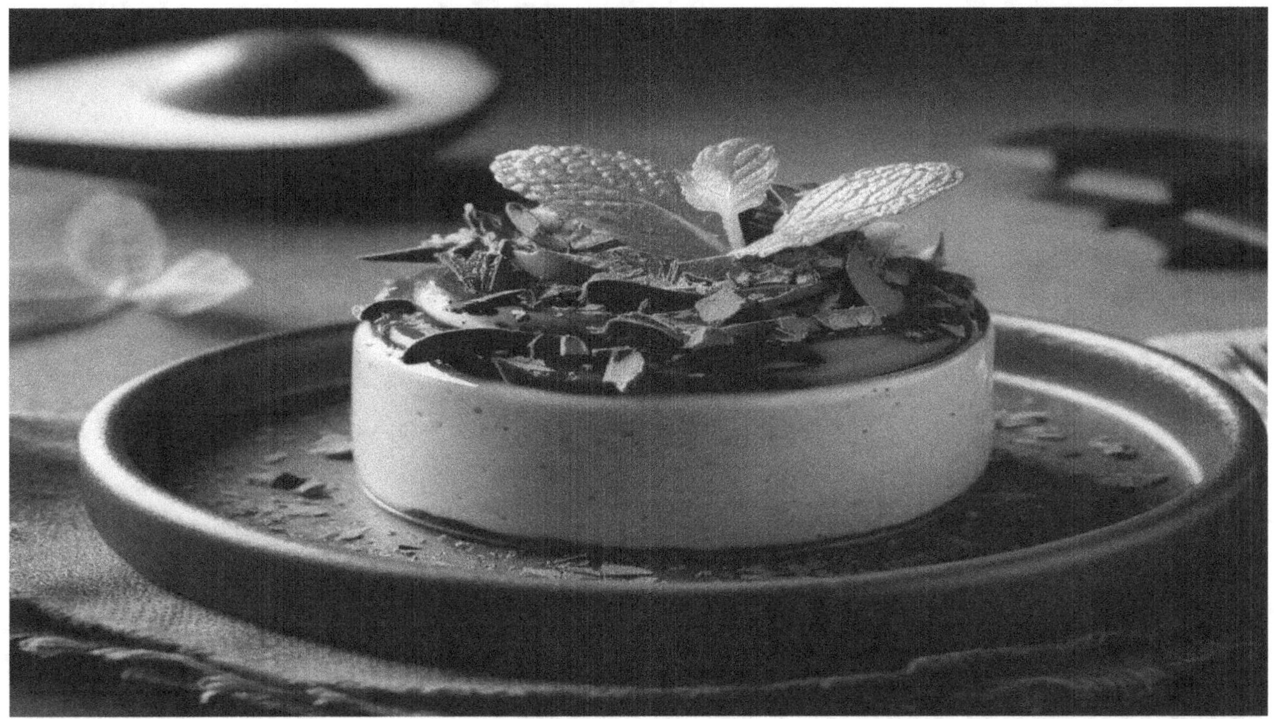

Dark Chocolate Avocado Mousse

Nutritional Information: Calories: 240, Protein: 3g, Carbohydrates: 30g, Fat: 15g, Fiber: 7g, Sodium: 10mg.

Ingredients:

- 2 ripe avocados, peeled and pitted
- 1/4 cup cocoa powder
- 1/4 cup honey
- 1 teaspoon vanilla extract
- Shaved chocolate and mint for garnish

Prep Time: 10 minutes, **Chill Time**: 1 hour, **Servings**: 4

Instructions:

1. Blend avocados, cocoa powder, honey, and vanilla until smooth.

2. Divide into serving dishes and chill for at least 1 hour.

3. Garnish with shaved chocolate and mint leaves before serving.

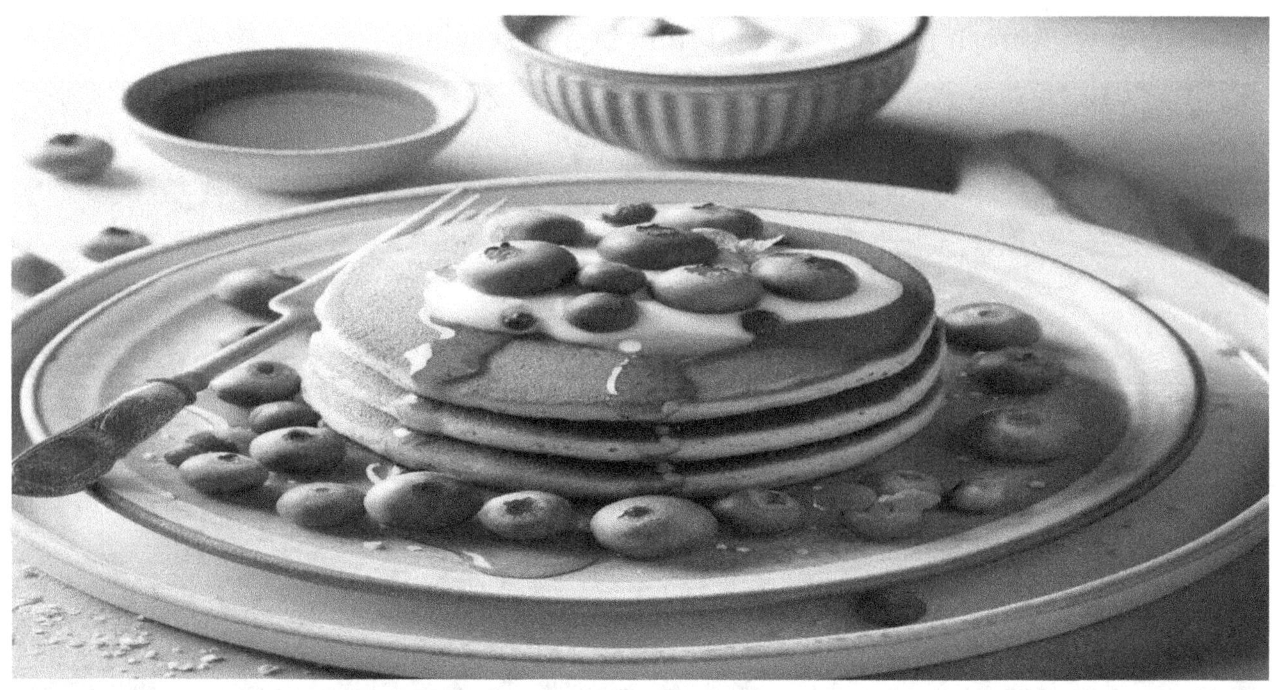

Coconut Flour Pancakes with Blueberries

Nutritional Information: Calories: 180, Protein: 6g, Carbohydrates: 20g, Fat: 10g, Fiber: 5g, Sodium: 150mg.

Ingredients:

- 1/2 cup coconut flour
- 1/2 teaspoon baking powder
- 2 eggs
- 1 cup almond milk
- 1 tablespoon maple syrup, plus extra for serving
- 1/2 cup blueberries
- Greek yogurt for serving

Prep Time: 10 minutes, **Cook Time**: 15 minutes, **Servings**: 4

Instructions:

1. Mix coconut flour and baking powder in a bowl.
2. In another bowl, whisk eggs, almond milk, and maple syrup. Add to dry ingredients and stir until combined.
3. Heat a non-stick skillet over medium heat and pour batter to form small pancakes.
4. Cook until bubbles form, then flip and cook until golden.

5. Serve pancakes with blueberries, a dollop of Greek yogurt, and drizzle with additional maple syrup.

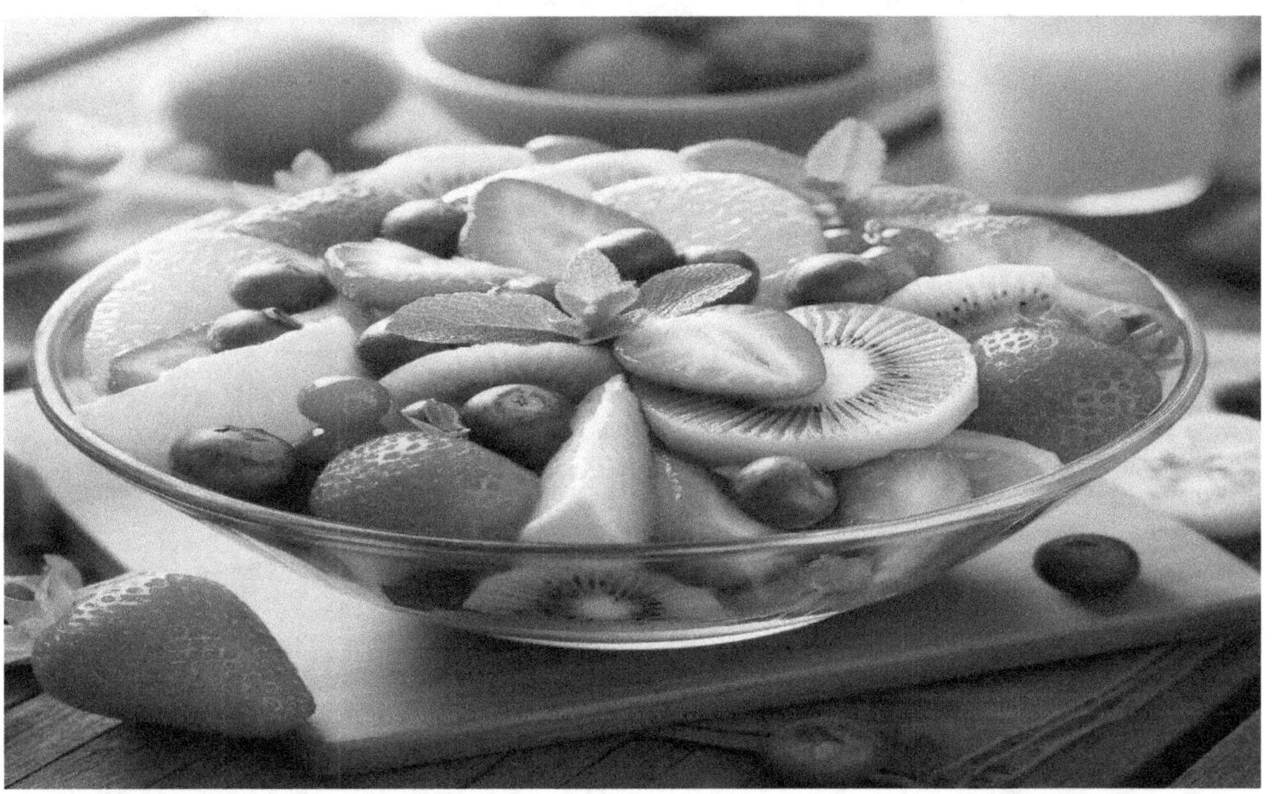

Colorful Fruit Salad

Nutritional Information: Calories: 90, Protein: 1g, Carbohydrates: 22g, Fat: 0.5g, Fiber: 4g, Sodium: 5mg.

Ingredients:

- 1 cup strawberries, sliced
- 1 kiwi, peeled and sliced
- 1 orange, peeled and segmented
- 1 cup blueberries
- Fresh mint leaves for garnish

Prep Time: 10 minutes, **Cook Time**: 0 minutes, **Servings**: 4

Instructions:

1. In a large bowl, combine all the sliced fruits.

2. Gently toss the fruits together.

3. Garnish with fresh mint leaves before serving.

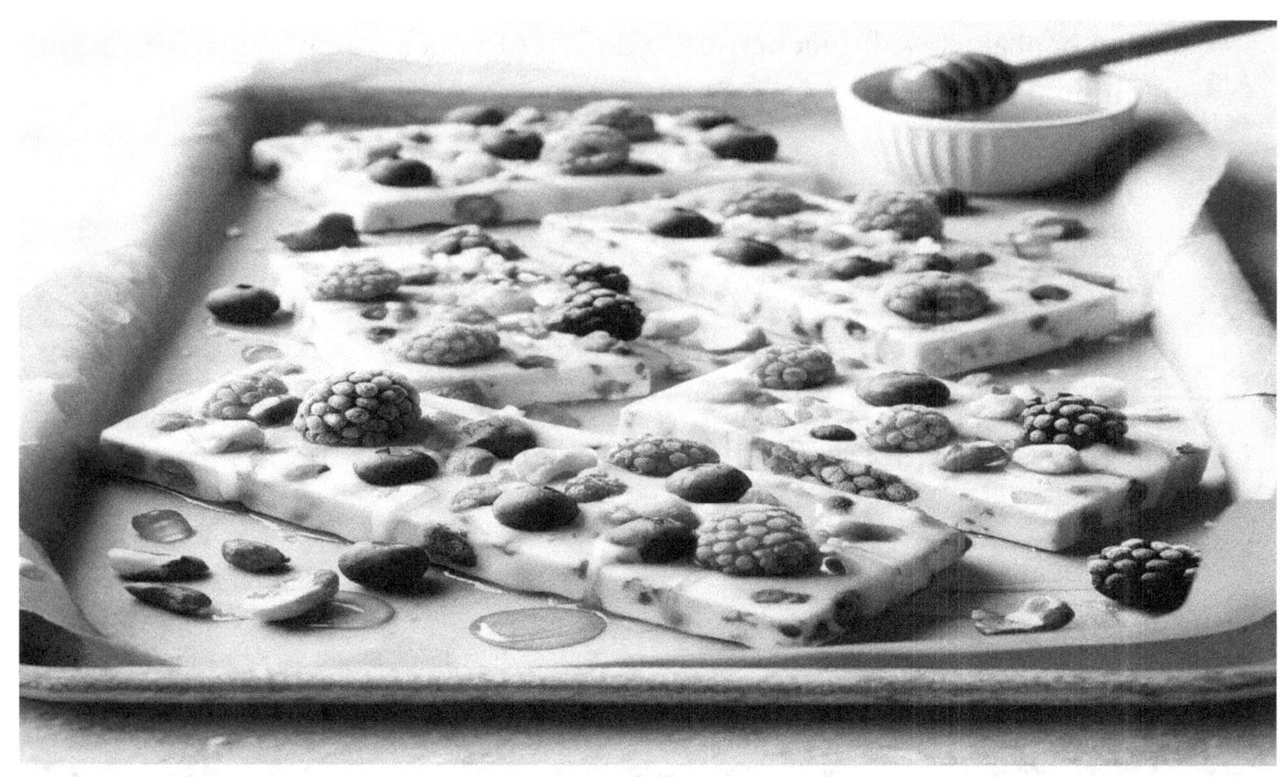

Frozen Yogurt Bark

Nutritional Information: Calories: 180, Protein: 10g, Carbohydrates: 18g, Fat: 8g, Fiber: 2g, Sodium: 45mg.

Ingredients:

- 2 cups Greek yogurt, plain
- 1/2 cup mixed berries (raspberries, blueberries)
- 1/4 cup chopped nuts (almonds, walnuts)
- 2 tablespoons honey

Prep Time: 5 minutes, **Freeze Time**: 2 hours, **Servings**: 4

Instructions:

1. Line a baking tray with parchment paper.
2. Spread Greek yogurt evenly on the tray.
3. Sprinkle mixed berries and chopped nuts over the yogurt.
4. Drizzle honey on top.
5. Freeze for at least 2 hours until firm. Break into pieces before serving.

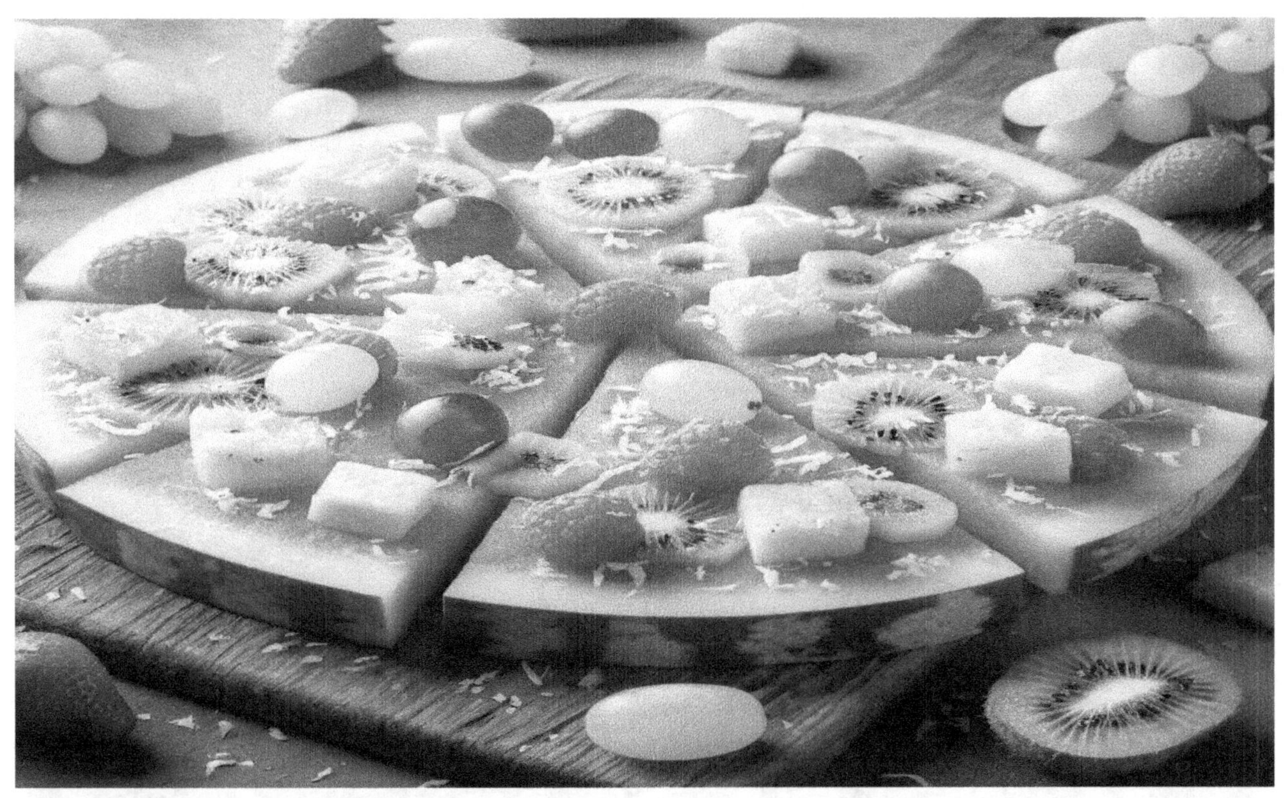

Watermelon Pizza

Nutritional Information: Calories: 70, Protein: 1g, Carbohydrates: 18g, Fat: 1g, Fiber: 2g, Sodium: 3mg.

Ingredients:

- 1 large slice of watermelon, cut into pizza-like slices
- 1/2 cup mixed fresh fruits (kiwi, pineapple, grapes)
- 1 tablespoon shredded coconut

Prep Time: 10 minutes, **Cook Time**: 0 minutes, **Servings**: 4

Instructions:

1. Place the large watermelon slice on a cutting board.
2. Arrange mixed fruits on top of the watermelon.
3. Sprinkle with shredded coconut.
4. Cut into pizza-like slices and serve.

Mini Fruit Tarts

Nutritional Information: Calories: 320, Protein: 6g, Carbohydrates: 45g, Fat: 15g, Fiber: 6g, Sodium: 15mg.

Ingredients:

- 1 cup dates, pitted
- 1/2 cup mixed nuts (almonds, walnuts)
- 1 cup cashews, soaked in water for 4 hours and drained
- 1/4 cup coconut milk
- 1 tablespoon honey
- 1/2 cup mixed fresh fruits (strawberries, kiwi, blueberries)

Prep Time: 20 minutes, **Chill Time**: 1 hour, **Servings**: 4

Instructions:

1. In a food processor, blend dates and nuts until they form a sticky dough. Press into mini tart pans to form the crust.

2. Blend cashews, coconut milk, and honey until smooth for the filling.

3. Spoon the filling into each tart crust.

4. Top with sliced fresh fruits.

5. Chill in the refrigerator for at least 1 hour before serving.

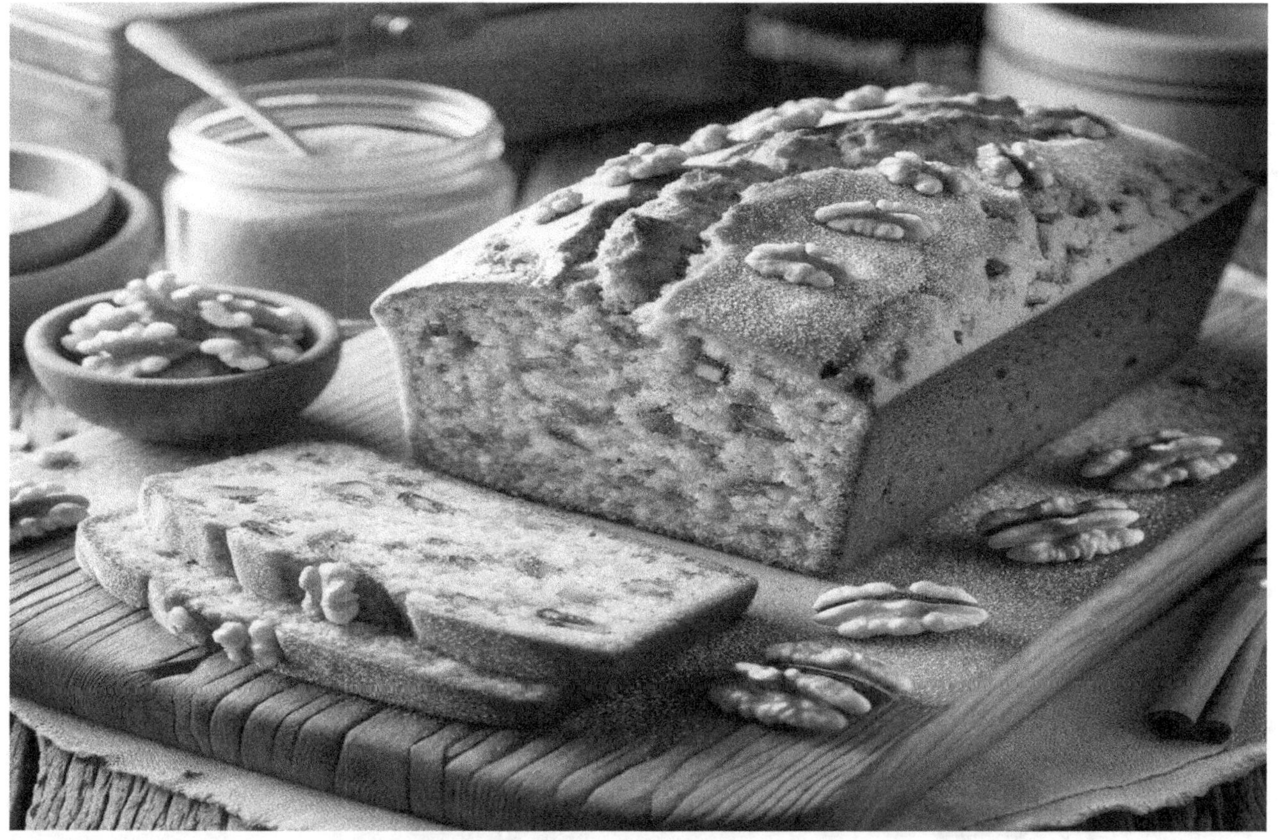

Whole Grain Banana Walnut Bread

Nutritional Information: Calories: 270, Protein: 6g, Carbohydrates: 44g, Fat: 9g, Fiber: 5g, Sodium: 300mg.

Ingredients:

- 2 cups whole wheat flour
- 3 ripe bananas, mashed
- 1/2 cup walnuts, chopped
- 1/3 cup honey
- 1/4 cup unsweetened applesauce
- 2 eggs
- 1 teaspoon vanilla extract
- 1 teaspoon baking soda
- 1/2 teaspoon salt
- 1/2 teaspoon cinnamon

Prep Time: 10 minutes, **Bake Time**: 45 minutes, **Servings**: 8

Instructions:

1. Preheat oven to 350°F (175°C). Grease a loaf pan.

2. In a large bowl, mix flour, baking soda, salt, and cinnamon.

3. In another bowl, whisk together mashed bananas, honey, applesauce, eggs, and vanilla.

4. Stir the wet ingredients into the dry until just combined. Fold in walnuts.

5. Pour batter into the prepared pan. Bake for 45 minutes or until a toothpick inserted in the center comes out clean.

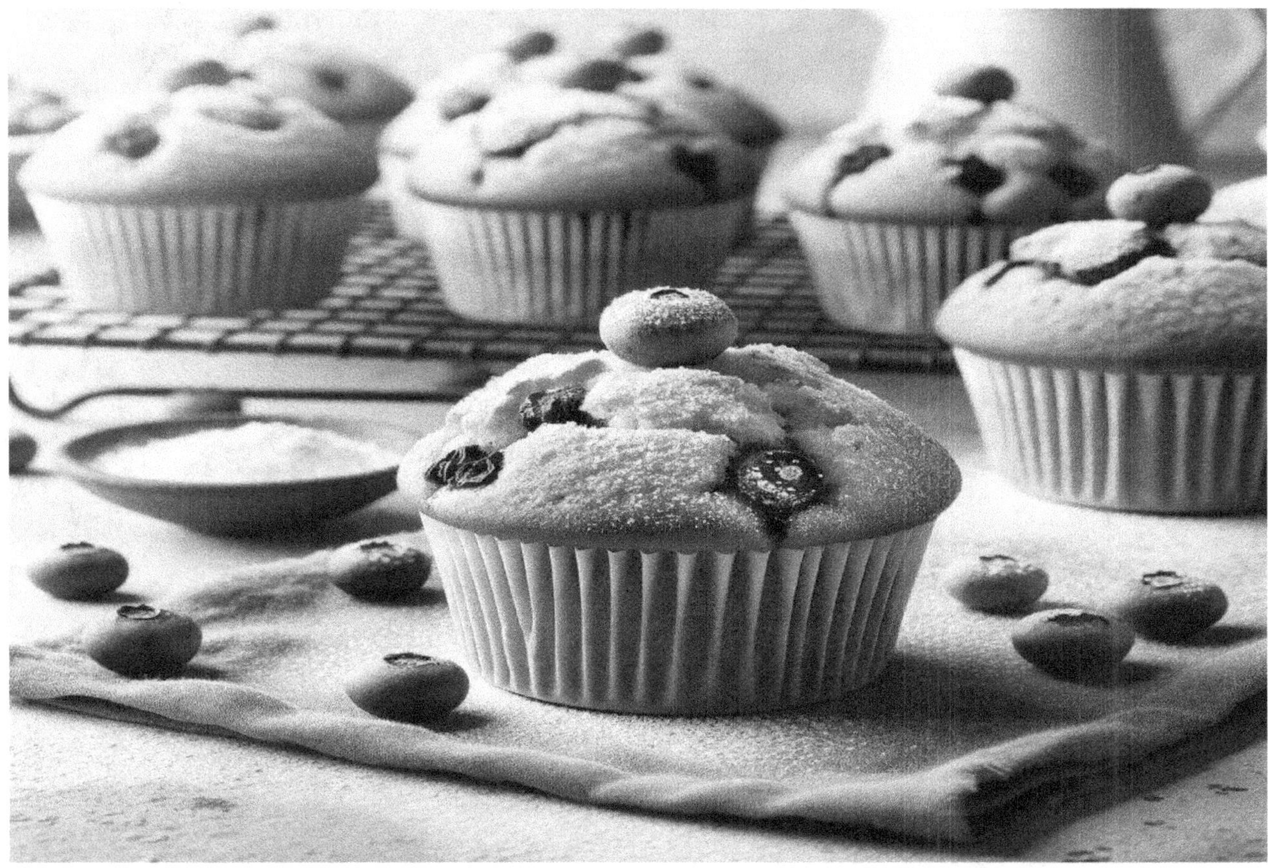

Gluten-Free Almond Flour Blueberry Muffins

Nutritional Information: Calories: 160, Protein: 6g, Carbohydrates: 12g, Fat: 11g, Fiber: 3g, Sodium: 80mg.

Ingredients:

- 2 cups almond flour
- 1/2 cup blueberries
- 1/4 cup honey
- 3 eggs

- 1/3 cup unsweetened almond milk
- 1 teaspoon baking powder
- 1/2 teaspoon vanilla extract
- Pinch of salt

Prep Time: 15 minutes, **Bake Time**: 25 minutes, **Servings**: 12

Instructions:

1. Preheat oven to 350°F (175°C). Line a muffin tin with paper liners.

2. In a bowl, combine almond flour, baking powder, and salt.

3. In another bowl, whisk eggs, almond milk, honey, and vanilla.

4. Mix wet ingredients into dry ingredients until combined. Fold in blueberries.

5. Divide batter among muffin cups. Bake for 25 minutes or until golden and a toothpick comes out clean.

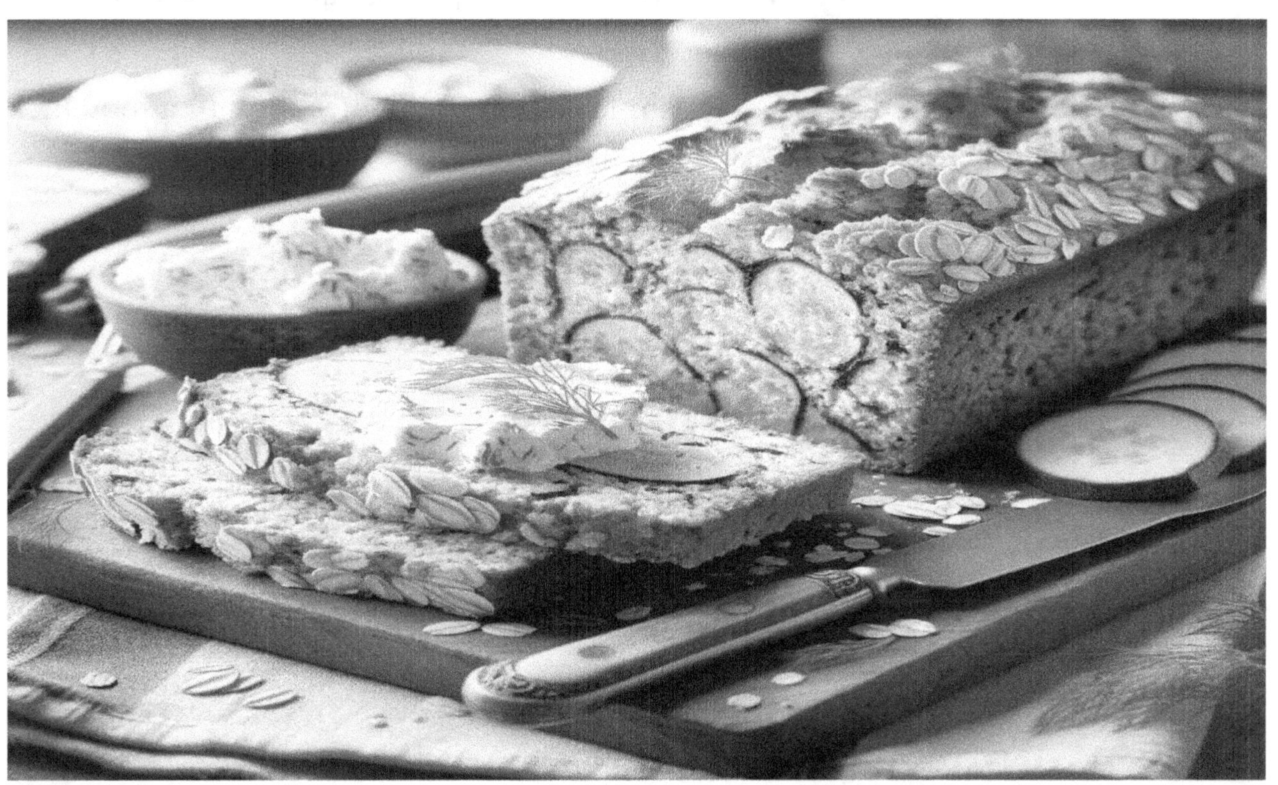

Savory Oat and Zucchini Bread

Nutritional Information: Calories: 210, Protein: 6g, Carbohydrates: 27g, Fat: 9g, Fiber: 4g, Sodium: 200mg.

Ingredients:

- 2 cups rolled oats
- 1 large zucchini, grated
- 1/2 cup low-fat milk
- 2 eggs
- 1/4 cup olive oil
- 2 tablespoons herbed cream cheese
- 1 teaspoon baking powder
- Salt and pepper to taste

Prep Time: 20 minutes, **Bake Time**: 40 minutes, **Servings**: 8

Instructions:

1. Preheat oven to 375°F (190°C). Grease a loaf pan.
2. In a bowl, combine oats, baking powder, salt, and pepper.
3. In another bowl, mix milk, eggs, olive oil, and cream cheese.
4. Stir wet ingredients into dry ingredients until just combined. Fold in grated zucchini.
5. Pour mixture into the prepared pan. Bake for 40 minutes or until a toothpick inserted comes out clean.

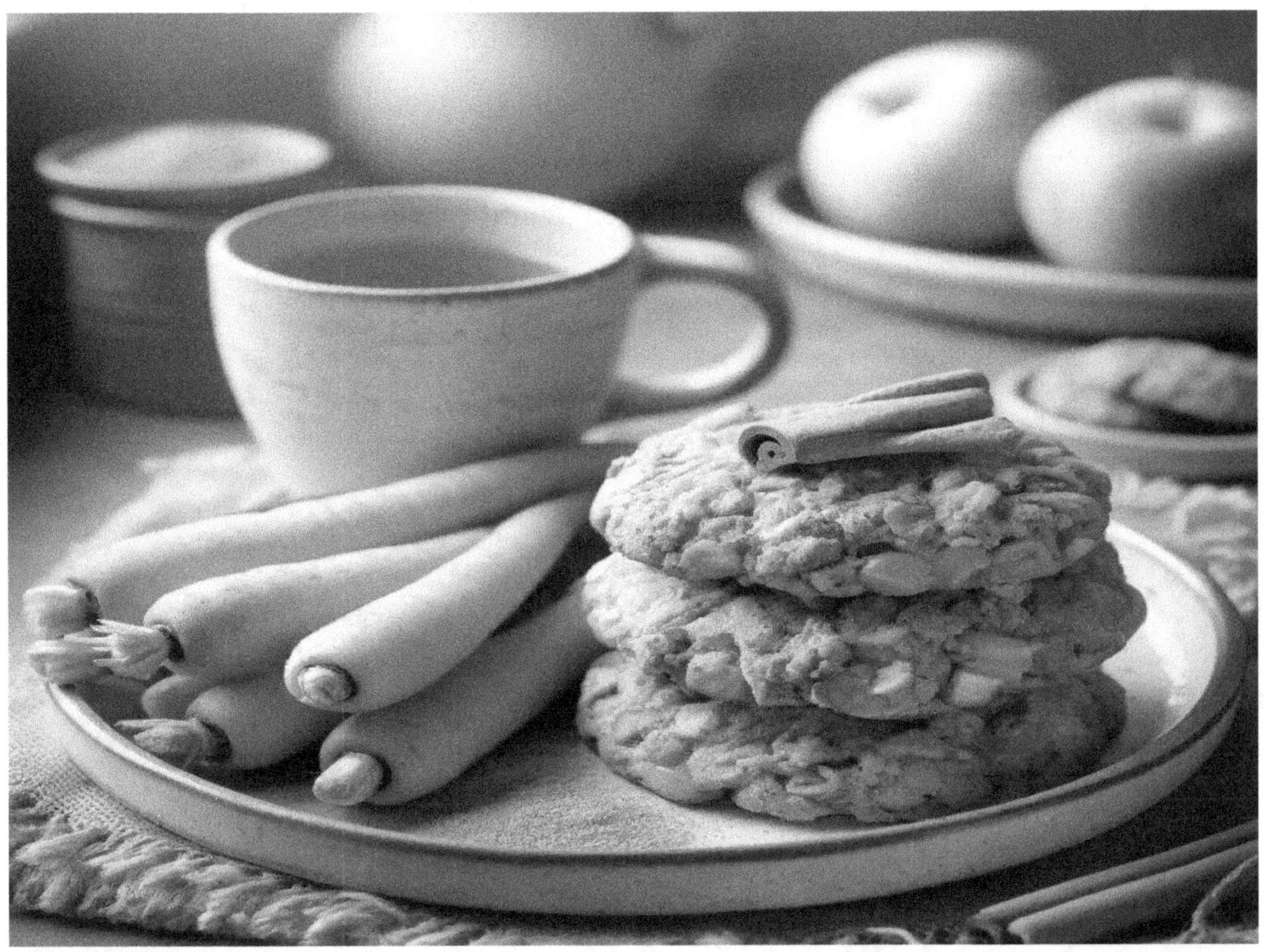

Carrot and Apple Fiber-Rich Cookies

Nutritional Information: Calories: 110, Protein: 2g, Carbohydrates: 18g, Fat: 4g, Fiber: 2g, Sodium: 55mg.

Ingredients:

- 1 cup grated carrots
- 1 cup grated apples
- 1/2 cup rolled oats
- 1/2 cup whole wheat flour
- 1/4 cup honey
- 1 egg
- 1/4 cup unsalted butter, melted
- 1 teaspoon cinnamon
- 1/2 teaspoon baking soda

Prep Time: 15 minutes, **Bake Time**: 15 minutes, **Servings**: 12

Instructions:

1. Preheat oven to 350°F (175°C). Line a baking sheet with parchment paper.

2. In a bowl, mix flour, oats, cinnamon, and baking soda.

3. In another bowl, combine honey, egg, and melted butter. Stir in carrots and apples.

4. Mix wet ingredients into dry ingredients until combined.

5. Drop tablespoonfuls of the dough onto the prepared baking sheet. Bake for 15 minutes or until edges are golden.

S/N	BREAKFAST	LUNCH	DINNER	SNACKS
DAY 1	Green Detox Smoothie	Grilled Chicken Caesar Wrap	Chicken and Vegetable Stir-Fry	Homemade Trail Mix
DAY 2	Berry Antioxidant Smoothie	Mediterranean Veggie Sandwich	Turkey Chili	Banana Kiwi Smoothie Bowl
DAY 3	Tropical Digestive Aid Smoothie	Avocado and Tomato Crackers	Seafood Paella	Greek Yogurt with Granola and Blueberries
DAY 4	Carrot Ginger Detox Juice	Whole Grain Banana Walnut Bread	Lentil and Sweet Potato Stew	Watermelon Pizza
DAY 5	Coconut Flour Pancakes	Savory Oat and Zucchini Bread	Baked Apples	Creamy Avocado Hummus
DAY 6	Mini Fruit Tarts	Spicy Black Bean Dip	Steamed Green Beans with Almonds	Frozen Yogurt Bark

DAY 7	No-Bake Cheesecake with Raspberries	Colorful Quinoa Salad	Roasted Brussels Sprouts with Garlic	Dark Chocolate Avocado Mousse
DAY 8	Green Detox Smoothie	Grilled Chicken Caesar Wrap	Gluten-Free Almond Flour Blueberry Muffins	Homemade Trail Mix
DAY 9	Berry Antioxidant Smoothie	Mediterranean Veggie Sandwich	Turkey Chili	Banana Kiwi Smoothie Bowl
DAY 10	Tropical Digestive Aid Smoothie	Avocado and Tomato Crackers	Seafood Paella	Greek Yogurt with Granola and Blueberries
DAY 11	Carrot Ginger Detox Juice	Whole Grain Banana Walnut Bread	Lentil and Sweet Potato Stew	Watermelon Pizza
DAY 12	Coconut Flour Pancakes	Savory Oat and Zucchini Bread	Baked Apples	Creamy Avocado Hummus

DAY 13	Mini Fruit Tarts	Spicy Black Bean Dip	Steamed Green Beans with Almonds	Frozen Yogurt Bark
DAY 14	Spinach and Mushroom Egg Muffins	Colorful Quinoa Salad	Roasted Brussels Sprouts with Garlic	Dark Chocolate Avocado Mousse
DAY 15	Green Detox Smoothie	Grilled Chicken Caesar Wrap	Gluten-Free Almond Flour Blueberry Muffins	Homemade Trail Mix
DAY 17	Tropical Digestive Aid Smoothie	Avocado and Tomato Crackers	Seafood Paella	Greek Yogurt with Granola and Blueberries
DAY 18	Carrot Ginger Detox Juice	Whole Grain Banana Walnut Bread	Lentil and Sweet Potato Stew	Watermelon Pizza
DAY 19	Coconut Flour Pancakes	Savory Oat and Zucchini Bread	Baked Apples	Creamy Avocado Hummus

DAY 20	Mini Fruit Tarts	Spicy Black Bean Dip	Steamed Green Beans with Almonds	Frozen Yogurt Bark
DAY 21	No-Bake Cheesecake with Raspberries	Colorful Quinoa Salad	Roasted Brussels Sprouts with Garlic	Dark Chocolate Avocado Mousse
DAY 22	Green Detox Smoothie	Grilled Chicken Caesar Wrap	Gluten-Free Almond Flour Blueberry Muffins	Homemade Trail Mix
DAY 23	Berry Antioxidant Smoothie	Mediterranean Veggie Sandwich	Turkey Chili	Banana Kiwi Smoothie Bowl
DAY 24	Spinach and Mushroom Egg Muffins	Avocado and Tomato Crackers	Seafood Paella	Greek Yogurt with Granola and Blueberries
DAY 25	Carrot Ginger Detox Juice	Whole Grain Banana Walnut Bread	Lentil and Sweet Potato Stew	Watermelon Pizza

DAY 26	Coconut Flour Pancakes	Savory Oat and Zucchini Bread	Baked Apples	Creamy Avocado Hummus
DAY 27	Mini Fruit Tarts	Spicy Black Bean Dip	Steamed Green Beans with Almonds	Frozen Yogurt Bark
Day 28	No-Bake Cheesecake with Raspberries	Colorful Quinoa Salad	Roasted Brussels Sprouts with Garlic,	Dark Chocolate Avocado Mousse
DAY 29	Green Detox Smoothie	Grilled Chicken Caesar Wrap	Turkey Chili	Homemade Trail Mix
DAY 30	Berry Antioxidant Smoothie	Mediterranean Veggie Sandwich	Seafood Paella	Banana Kiwi Smoothie Bowl

Meal Planning Tips and Strategies

Meal preparation plays a pivotal role in promoting a healthy diet, particularly for individuals who are tasked with managing particular health conditions, such as non-alcoholic fatty liver disease. Meal planning plays a dual role: it facilitates adherence to dietary guidelines and reduces the daily burden associated with meal selection, thereby promoting portion control and the maintenance of a well-balanced diet. The following are pragmatic advice and approaches to assist novices in developing a dietary plan that promotes liver health and holistic well-being.

A Fundamental Comprehension of Meal Planning

Meal planning entails the selection of meals for a specified time period, such as a month or a week. It additionally entails selecting ingredients, determining the recipes, and occasionally pre-planning meals. The objective is to optimize the culinary procedure, minimize food wastage, and guarantee adherence to a nourishing dietary regimen.

1. Begin with a Weekly Strategy

For novices, a weekly diet plan is more feasible and less intimidating. It offers sufficient adaptability to accommodate social obligations or alterations in one's timetable. Start by choosing meals for various periods of the day — breakfast, lunch, supper, and snacks. Incorporate a diversity of foods to cover all dietary categories, ensuring that each meal is balanced with proteins, carbohydrates, and fats.

2. Inventory Your Kitchen

Check your larder, freezer, and fridge to see what ingredients you already have. It helps prevent overbuying and lets you use what you already possess, reducing food waste and saving money. Use these ingredients to discuss meal ideas or search for recipes that utilize them.

3. Choose Recipes Wisely

Select recipes based on their nutritional value, simplicity of preparation, and compatibility with your health objectives. For someone with NAFLD, focus on recipes that are low in saturated fats and sugars but high in fiber and healthy lipids. Think grilled fish, steamed vegetables, and salads rich in verdant greens. It's also beneficial to choose recipes that can be prepared in bulk and stored, such as soups, stews, and casseroles.

4. Create a Shopping List

Once your meals are selected, compile a purchasing list. Organize this list by categories such as vegetables, fruits, dairy, and proteins to expedite your shopping excursion. Stick to your list to avoid impulse buys that might not work into your dietary plan.

5. Prep in Advance

Meal preparation can save significant time during the week. Dedicate a few hours over the weekend to mince vegetables, marinate proteins, or even prepare meals in advance. Store prepared ingredients in clear containers in the refrigerator to keep them fresh and visible.

6. Portion Control

When preparing dishes, consider portion proportions. Using measuring containers or a kitchen scale can help manage portions effectively, ensuring you do not overspend. This is particularly crucial in a diet for NAFLD, where managing caloric intake can help control the disease's progression.

7. Flexible and Forgiving

Your dietary plan should have flexibility. If a meal doesn't happen as planned, it's acceptable to swap it with another day's meal or use readily available ingredients to create something simple. The key is to avoid opting for harmful choices because your plan feels too rigid.

8. Monitor and Adjust

Keep track of what meals worked well and which didn't. Maybe some recipes were too complex, or you found certain dishes didn't agree with you. Adjust your plan based on this feedback. Meal planning is an evolving process that conforms to your lifestyle, taste preferences, and health requirements.

Tools and Resources

To assist with meal planning, many instruments are available. Digital applications can help construct grocery lists, discover recipes, and monitor your nutritional intake. Websites offer meal planning templates and planners that can be printed for simple reference.

Benefits Beyond Diet

Beyond increasing diet quality, meal planning can enhance your understanding of nutrition and its effects on the body. It encourages cooking at home, which is typically healthier than dining out. Financially, it helps budget food expenses more effectively. Psychologically, it reduces mealtime anxiety and decision fatigue, contributing to a more structured and stress-free day.

Meal planning isn't just about following a diet; it's about creating a sustainable lifestyle that promotes health and well-being. With practice, it becomes a natural part of your weekly regimen, resulting to lasting benefits for both your liver health and overall lifestyle.

CHAPTER 10: THE SCIENCE OF SUPPLEMENTS

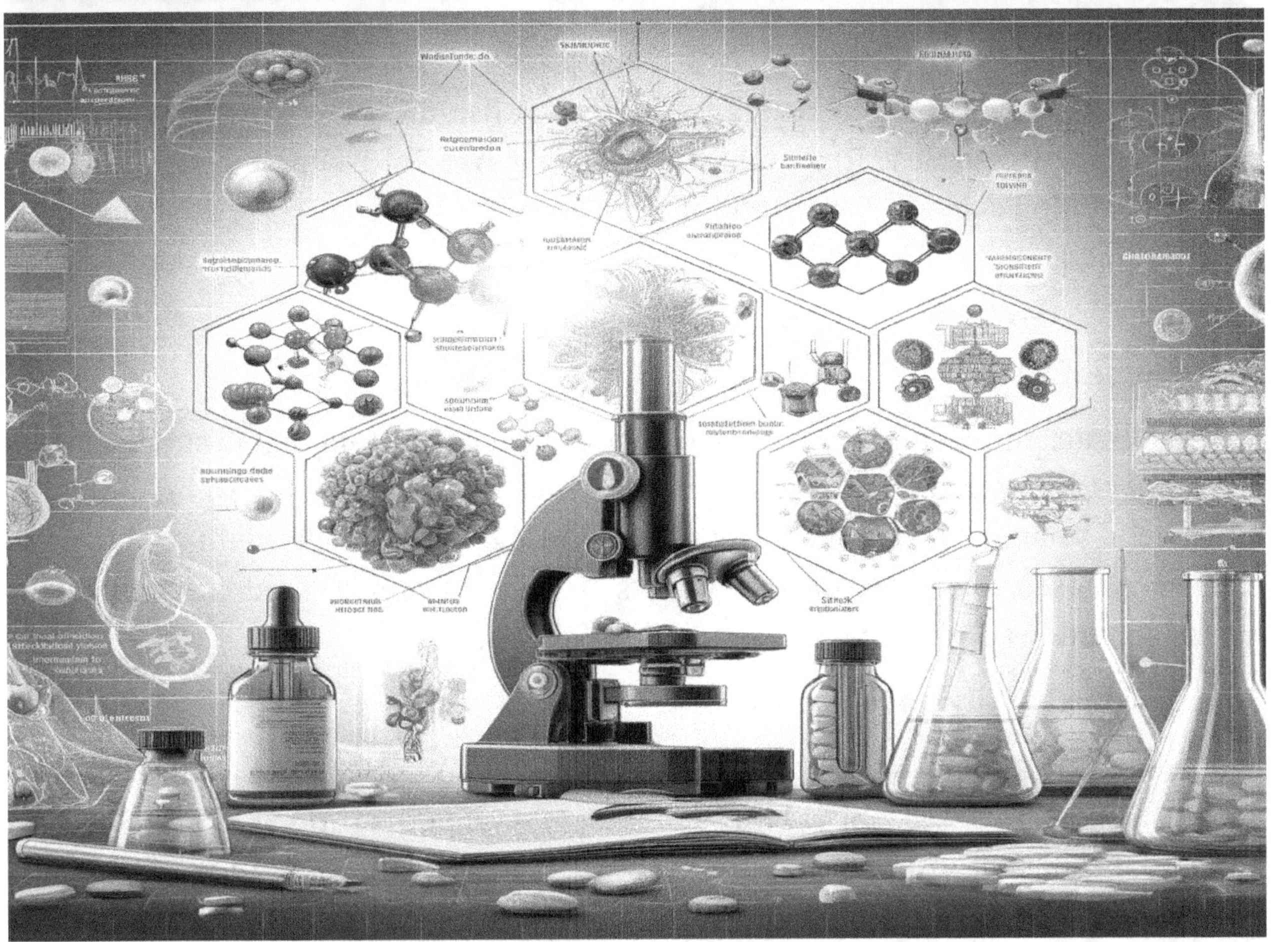

Supplements and NAFLD: What Works and What Doesn't

When managing Non-Alcoholic Fatty Liver Disease (NAFLD), the cornerstone of treatment typically involves diet and lifestyle modifications. However, the function of dietary supplements in managing this condition is a topic of interest for many. It's crucial to understand what supplements may offer benefits and which ones might not be effective, or even potentially hazardous. This discussion seeks to provide a clear overview of the current understanding of supplements in the context of NAFLD.

Understanding Supplements for NAFLD

Supplements are often considered as an aid to enhance liver health, particularly when dietary intake might fall short. For individuals with NAFLD, certain supplements have been investigated for their prospective liver benefits.

1. Omega-3 Fatty Acids

Omega-3 fatty acids, particularly those present in fish oil, are known for their anti-inflammatory properties. Research suggests that omega-3 supplements can help reduce liver lipids and inflammation in persons with NAFLD. They are considered harmless and might aid in lowering elevated liver enzymes, a common issue in NAFLD.

2. Vitamin E

Vitamin E, an antioxidant, has been shown to enhance liver function in some patients with NAFLD by reducing oxidative stress and inflammation within the liver. However, Vitamin E supplementation should be approached with caution, as excessive doses can have adverse effects, particularly in individuals with other health conditions or those taking certain medications.

3. Milk Thistle (Silymarin)

Milk thistle is a supplement often used for its potential to protect the liver and enhance liver function. Silymarin, an active component of milk thistle, has antioxidant and anti-inflammatory properties. Studies have shown conflicting results regarding its effectiveness in treating NAFLD, and it is generally considered safe for most individuals.

4. Vitamin D

A deficiency in vitamin D is common in individuals with NAFLD, and there is emerging evidence that vitamin D supplementation might help enhance liver function in NAFLD patients. More research is required to confirm these findings, but ensuring adequate vitamin D levels is important for overall health.

5. Probiotics

The gut-liver axis plays a significant role in the development and progression of NAFLD. Probiotics can influence gastrointestinal health and, by extension, may benefit liver health by reducing intestinal permeability and bacterial translocation.

Clinical trials suggest that probiotics may reduce liver enzymes and inflammation in NAFLD patients.

What Doesn't Work

While some supplements show promise, others do not have substantial evidence to support their efficacy in NAFLD management or may be detrimental.

1. Unproven Herbal Supplements

Many herbal supplements claim to enhance liver health but lack clinical evidence. Some might even cause harm. For instance, supplements like kava and comfrey have been linked to liver harm. Always consult healthcare providers before commencing any new supplement, especially herbal ones.

2. Weight Loss Pills and Over-the-Counter Medications

Non-prescription weight loss drugs and certain over-the-counter medications may worsen liver health and should be avoided by those with NAFLD. These products can burden the liver, leading to increased liver fat or liver injury.

General Advice on Supplements

- **Consultation:** Always consult a healthcare provider before commencing any supplements, particularly if you have NAFLD or other health conditions. This ensures safety and appropriateness of the supplement for your specific health requirements.
- **Regulation:** Understand that supplements are not regulated as strictly as medications, which means their integrity and potency can vary. Opt for supplements that have been third-party tested for quality and accuracy in labeling.
- **Holistic Approach:** Supplements should not supplant a healthy diet and lifestyle adjustments. They should be used to complement dietary efforts aimed at enhancing liver health.

Safe Supplement Practices for Liver Health

Understanding and implementing safe supplement practices is crucial, particularly when it comes to maintaining liver health. The liver plays a central function in processing everything we ingest, including food, beverages, and dietary supplements. Therefore, knowing how to choose and use supplements safely is essential to preventing liver injury and supporting overall liver function. This guide will provide novices with essential information on safe supplement practices tailored specifically for enhancing liver health.

Introduction to Dietary Supplements

Dietary supplements include vitamins, minerals, botanicals, amino acids, and enzymes marketed in various forms such as capsules, granules, and liquids. They are intended to supplement the diet and offer nutritional benefits. However, supplements are not intended to replace comprehensive meals which provide the nutritional balance essential for health. It's also essential to note that supplements are regulated as food, not as drugs, which means they do not endure the rigorous testing that medications do for efficacy and safety.

Choosing the Right Supplements

1. Research Before You Buy

Investigate the benefits and potential adverse effects of any supplement before consuming it. Reliable sources include academic journals, credible health websites, and consultations with healthcare professionals.

2. Quality Over Quantity

Opt for high-quality brands that voluntarily submit their products for testing by independent organizations like US Pharmacopeia (USP), ConsumerLab, or NSF International.

3. Understand Supplement Labels

Read and understand everything on the supplement label, including the serving size, volume, and active constituents. Pay heed to the "% Daily Value" to ensure you're not consuming too much.

Integrating Supplements into Your Diet

1. Start with a Food-First Approach

Prioritize obtaining your nutrients from a balanced diet. Use supplements to cover voids but not as a substitute for a diverse diet.

2. Consult Healthcare Providers

Always consult with a healthcare provider before starting new supplements, particularly if you have existing health conditions or you're taking other medications. This prevents potential negative interactions and ensures the supplement is appropriate for your specific health requirements.

3. Keep Track of What You Take

Maintain a list of all the supplements you use and the dosages. This information can be crucial for your healthcare provider to manage your overall treatment plan and avoid interactions.

Safe Usage of Supplements

1. Follow Recommended Doses

Stick to the recommended doses unless otherwise directed by a healthcare professional. High quantities of certain vitamins and minerals can cause health problems, including serious liver injury.

2. Monitor Your Body's Response

Pay heed to your body's reactions after commencing a supplement. If you experience any adverse effects, such as nausea, dizziness, rapid pulse, or peculiar fatigue, cease taking the supplement and consult your healthcare provider immediately.

3. Regular Liver Function Tests

If you're taking supplements that can impact liver health, such as Vitamin A, niacin, or iron, regular liver function tests can help monitor the effects and prevent liver injury.

Special Considerations for Liver Health

1. Avoid Potentially Harmful Supplements

Some supplements are known to be detrimental to the liver. For example, avoid excessive quantities of Vitamin A and iron. Herbs like kava and comfrey have been linked to severe liver injury and should be avoided.

2. Supplements Known to Support Liver Health

Certain supplements may support liver health. Milk thistle, known for its silymarin content, can protect liver cells from injury and enhance function. Omega-3 fatty acids from fish oil are known to reduce liver obesity and inflammation in those with NAFLD.

3. Beware of Alcohol

If consuming alcohol, be extra cautious with supplements as the combination can impair liver function. Always seek advice from a healthcare provider on safe consumption patterns, particularly if liver health is a concern.

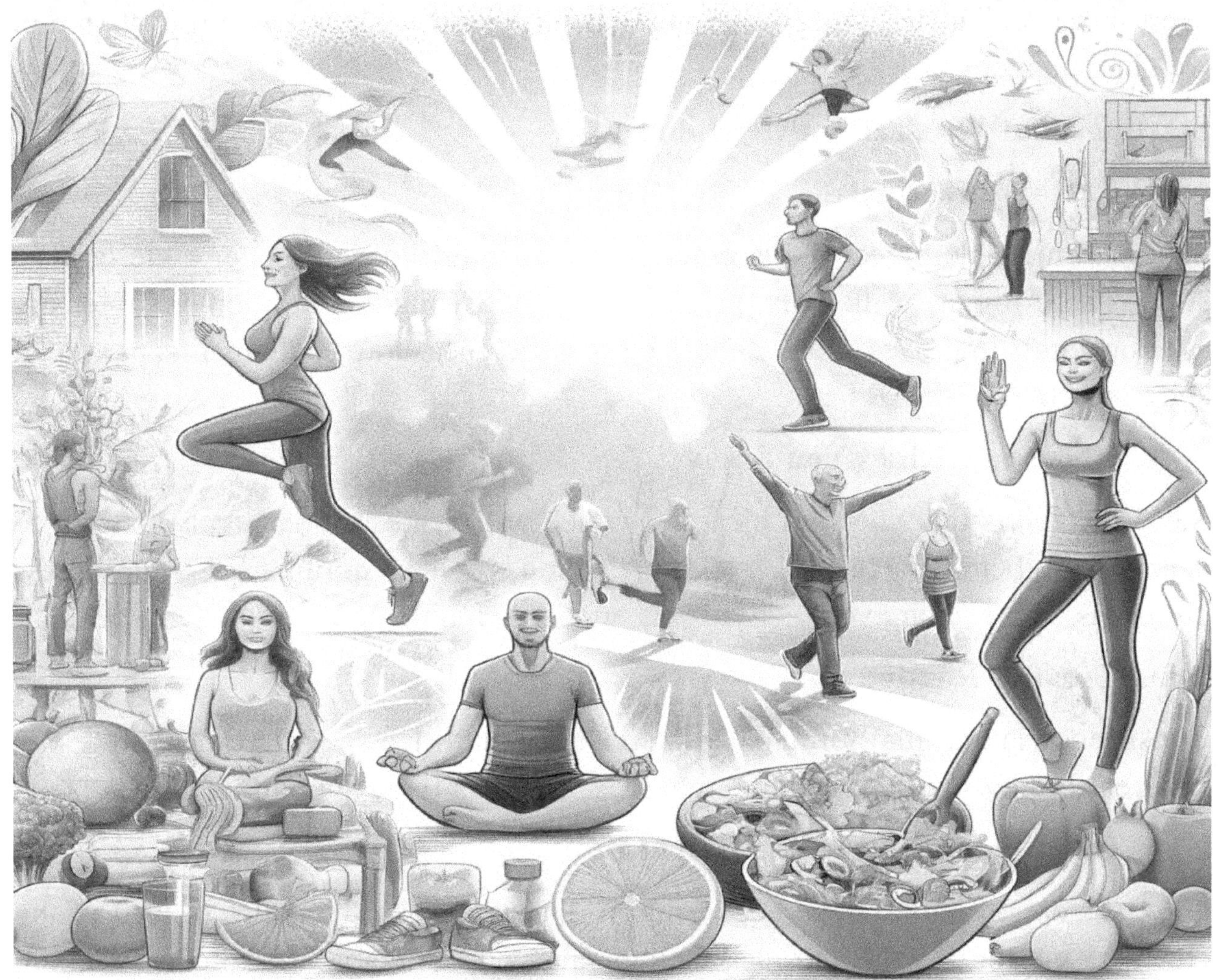

Incorporating Physical Activity into Your Routine

Incorporating physical activity into your daily regimen is a fundamental aspect of maintaining a wholesome lifestyle. For novices, the idea of integrating regular exercise can seem daunting. However, the benefits of regular physical activity are immense, not only for physical health but also for mental well-being. This guide provides essential tips and strategies for beginners on how to effectively implement exercise into their lives, enhancing the benefits of a nutritious diet, such as those enumerated in recipes throughout this cookbook.

Understanding the Importance of Physical Activity

Physical activity is crucial for maintaining a healthy weight, improving cardiovascular health, enhancing muscle strength, and bolstering mental health. Regular exercise helps manage tension, reduce the risk of chronic diseases such as heart disease, diabetes, and certain malignancies, and it plays a significant role in weight management.

Starting Your Physical Activity Journey

1. Set Realistic Goals

Setting achievable objectives is essential. Start with modest, manageable targets, such as a 10-minute walk daily, progressively increasing the duration and intensity as your fitness improves. Goals should be specific, measurable, attainable, pertinent, and time-bound (SMART).

2. Choose Activities You Enjoy

Select exercises that you find pleasant, which will make it more likely for you to persist with them. Whether it's walking, cycling, yoga, swimming, or group fitness programs, appreciating your activities is crucial to maintaining regular exercise.

3. Create a Routine

Consistency is essential for making exercise a habit. Plan specific times in the day or week for physical activity, and treat these times as fixed appointments.

4. Build Activity into Your Daily Life

Look for opportunities to be active during the day. Take the stairs instead of the elevator, go for a walk during lunch breaks, and attempt standing or walking meetings.

Overcoming Barriers to Exercise

1. Time Management

Many individuals believe they are too busy to squeeze in exercise. However, dividing up exercise into smaller segments throughout the day can be effective. Three 10-minute treks can be just as beneficial as one 30-minute walk.

2. Lack of Motivation

Stay motivated by keeping your routines varied and intriguing. Tracking your progress, setting challenges, and rewarding yourself when you reach your objectives can also help maintain motivation.

3. Physical Limitations

If you have physical limitations or medical concerns, consult with a healthcare provider or a fitness professional to devise a safe and effective exercise program tailored to your requirements.

Equipment and Space

1. Use What You Have

You don't necessarily need expensive apparatus or a gym membership to remain active. Many exercises require minimal or no apparatus, such as body-weight exercises like push-ups, sit-ups, and yoga.

2. Utilize Space Efficiently

Any tiny, clear area in your residence can serve as a workout space for activities like stretching or yoga. For more vigorous activities, a nearby park or recreational area can be a wonderful option.

Monitoring Your Progress

1. Track Your Activities

Keeping a record of your physical activities can help you remain on track and see how much you've accomplished over time. Use a notebook, an app, or a wearable device to monitor your progress.

2. Listen to Your Body

Pay attention to how your body feels during and after exercise. Some discomfort after physical activity is normal, but persistent or sharp pain is a sign that you may be pressing too hard.

3. Adjust as Needed

As you get fitter, your body will become more efficient at exercising. Regularly review and adjust your objectives and activities to keep challenging your body and progressing towards improved health.

Stress management is not only good for your mental health; it also helps to keep your liver healthy. Stress reduction might be just as essential as nutritional control for those with Non-Alcoholic Fatty Liver Disease (NAFLD). Chronic stress has been shown to aggravate liver issues by increasing inflammation and changing metabolic responses. This article will cover excellent stress management practices that promote not just a calm mind but also a healthy liver.

The Relationship Between Stress and Liver Health

The liver is a strong organ that performs a variety of critical processes such as detoxification, protein synthesis, and chemical generation required for digesting. Stress disrupts the body's hormonal equilibrium, resulting in higher cortisol levels, which can increase liver strain and promote fat storage and inflammation.

Effective Stress Management Techniques

1. Regular Physical Activity

Physical activity is an effective stress reliever. Brisk walking, running, swimming, and cycling can considerably reduce cortisol levels, improve blood circulation, and boost general fitness, all of which assist to reduce liver fat and inflammation. Aim for at least 150 minutes of moderate-intensity aerobic exercise each week, with muscle-strengthening activities on two or more days.

2. Mindfulness & Meditation

Meditation, particularly mindfulness-based stress reduction (MBSR), helps to reduce anxiety and stress by focusing your attention on the present moment. Regular meditation has been demonstrated to lower the body's stress response and hence improve liver function. Starting with a few minutes every day might be helpful.

3. Balanced Diet

A diet high in antioxidants, vitamins, and minerals can help counteract the oxidative stress linked with mental stress. Leafy greens, berries, nuts, and seeds are essential for both brain and hepatic health. Incorporate meals that promote liver cleansing and minimize inflammation.

4. Adequate Sleep

Getting enough sleep is essential for managing stress. Sleep deprivation can intensify stress, resulting in higher cortisol levels, which can worsen liver inflammation and fat storage. Adults should strive for 7-9 hours of quality sleep each night, with a consistent sleep pattern.

5. Deep Breathing Exercises.

Deep breathing exercises can stimulate the parasympathetic nervous system, which regulates the relaxation response. Techniques such as diaphragmatic breathing, which focuses on extending the belly rather than the chest, can help alleviate stress and are simple to practice at any time.

6. Yoga

Yoga blends physical postures, breath control, and meditation to promote both mental and physical wellness. Yoga's mild stretches and postures can help relieve muscular tension, increase flexibility, and reduce stress, all of which boost liver function.

7. Cognitive Behavior Therapy (CBT)

CBT is a type of psychotherapy that assists people in altering negative thought patterns in order to transform their feelings and actions. CBT can give strategies to better handle stress triggers, lowering pressure on your body and liver.

8. Social Support

Maintaining strong relationships with friends and family may offer emotional support and minimize stress. Social interactions can promote the release of oxytocin, a natural stress reliever. This is especially essential since feeling supported may help to reduce worry and stress, both of which can have an influence on liver function.

9. Time Management

Effective time management may help you avoid feeling overwhelmed, which is a major source of stress for many people. Setting priorities, breaking down activities into smaller parts, and delegating duties may all help you manage stress at work and home.

10.Journaling

Writing down ideas and feelings may considerably reduce stress and improve clarity in difficult times. Regular journaling can help you manage stress more effectively and reduce the strain on your liver.

Integrating Stress Management into Your Daily Routine.

Incorporating these tactics into your everyday routine demands persistence and dedication. Begin by selecting one or two ways that are compatible with your lifestyle and personality. Regular practice is essential, since the advantages of stress management accumulate and become more apparent with time.

The Role of Sleep in Weight and Health Management

Sleep, which is sometimes disregarded in today's hectic environment, is critical for weight control and overall wellness. Understanding the importance of sleep is critical for anybody embarking on a healthier lifestyle. This section explains how good sleep may have a significant impact on your physical health, weight, and general well-being.

Understanding Sleep's Effect on Health

Sleep is as important to our bodies as eating, drinking, and breathing, and it is required to sustain fundamental biological processes. It controls mood, cognitive function, and physical health. Sleep has a significant role in weight management and overall wellness.

The Link Between Sleep and Metabolism

Sleep has a profound impact on metabolic functions, such as how our bodies metabolize glucose, regulate hormones, and convert food to energy. Inadequate sleep can impair these functions. Poor sleep, for example, can cause insulin resistance, a precursor to type 2 diabetes, as well as impact the hormones ghrelin and leptin, which regulate hunger. Ghrelin conveys hunger to the brain, whereas leptin communicates satiety. When you don't get enough sleep, your ghrelin levels rise while your leptin levels fall, causing you to crave more food.

Sleep and Calorie Intake

According to research, those who sleep for fewer than seven hours each night eat more calories the next day. A lack of sleep is connected with increased snacking and intake of high-carbohydrate meals. This is a common cycle in which weary people turn to high-energy meals heavy in sugar and fat to immediately alleviate their energy deficit.

Fatigue and Physical Activity.

Adequate sleep is vital for maintaining energy levels, which has a direct influence on motivation for physical activity. When you are well-rested, you are more inclined to exercise and participate in physical activities. In contrast, sleep deprivation can lead to a sedentary lifestyle, which increases the risk of weight gain and other health problems.

Strategies to Improve Sleep

Improving the quality and length of your sleep will help you manage your weight and health more effectively. Here are some ways to help:

1. **Regular Sleeping Schedule:** Go to bed and get up at the same hour every day, including on weekends. This constancy strengthens your body's sleep-wake cycle.
2. **Create A Bedtime Ritual:** Before bedtime, engage in calm, soothing activities such as reading a book, having a warm bath, or practicing relaxation techniques. Avoid activities that are exciting, stressful, or anxious.
3. **Optimize Your Sleeping Environment**: Make your bedroom suitable to sleeping. Invest on a comfortable mattress and pillows, keep the room cool, and remove any light or noise that may disrupt your sleep.
4. **Limit Your Exposure to Light.:** Melatonin is a naturally occurring hormone that regulates your sleep-wake cycle in response to light exposure. Spend time in natural light during the day and limit screen time at least one hour before bed to encourage melatonin synthesis.
5. **Watch What You Eat and Drink:** Avoid going to bed hungry or full. Avoid eating heavy or substantial meals within a few hours of bedtime. Also, avoid tobacco, coffee, and alcohol, as these can impair sleep.
6. **Exercise Regularly:** Physical activity might help you fall asleep sooner and sleep deeper—but avoid exercising too close to bedtime.
7. **Manage Worries:** Before going to bed, try to address any worries or concerns you may have. Write down what's on your mind and lay it away for tomorrow.

The Bigger Picture

Incorporating proper sleep habits into your daily routine will significantly boost your health management efforts. Sleep not only helps manage weight by altering hunger hormones and metabolism, but it also aids in bodily recovery and regeneration, promoting active lives and healthier eating habits.

Real-life tales from people who have made big dietary adjustments and experienced dramatic improvements in their liver health may be great motivators. Here are seven testimonies demonstrating the beneficial effects that dietary changes may have on liver function.

Testimonial 1: Sarah's Recovery Journey

"After being diagnosed with NAFLD, I felt completely overwhelmed. My doctor recommended dietary adjustments as a starting point for managing my illness. I concentrated on eating more leafy greens, lean meats, and avoiding processed sweets and fats. Within six months, my liver enzyme levels were improved, and I had dropped 20 pounds. It was a difficult process, but adjusting my dietary habits truly saved my life."

Testimonial 2: Mike's Way to Better Health

"I never imagined that altering what I ate would have such a significant impact on my health. After experiencing weariness and liver pain, I decided to change my diet by limiting alcohol intake and eating more healthy foods. My most recent liver tests revealed a considerable reduction in liver fat, and I've never felt better."

Testimonial 3: Linda's Success Story

"I began eating a diet high in omega-3s and antioxidants, employing dishes that included fish, almonds, and plenty of veggies. My doctor was pleased at how rapidly my liver function tests improved. This lifestyle adjustment has benefited not only my liver but also my entire health."

Testimonial 4: John's Transformation

"After being told my liver was at risk, I focused on fiber-rich foods and reduced sugar and refined carbs." The transition was difficult, but the end result was worthwhile. Six months later, my hepatologist was astounded at the improvement in my liver's health."

Testimonial 5: Emma's Rejuvenation

"Learning to create liver-healthy foods has been a struggle for me. I switched from fried to grilled items and ate more fruits and vegetables. My energy levels have skyrocketed, and my liver enzymes are now within normal limits. It's like having a fresh lease on life."

Testimonial 6: Alex's newfound wellness

"After struggling with obesity and liver issues, I switched to a plant-based diet." It was a radical adjustment, but the favorable influence on my liver health was clear at my next medical check-up. My doctor confirmed that the inflammation had greatly diminished, and I felt like a whole new person."

Testimonial 7: Rachel's Lifestyle Changes

"I was doubtful about how nutrition may affect my liver illness. However, after following a strict no-sugar, no-alcohol diet rich in lean meats and veggies, my most recent tests revealed significant improvement. My hepatologist was delighted, and I've discovered that food actually is medicine."

These examples demonstrate the effectiveness of diet adjustments in controlling and enhancing liver health. They depict not only the difficulties encountered, but also the victories attained, bringing hope and inspiration to those on similar roads. Their stories demonstrate that with determination and the appropriate dietary choices, it is possible to improve one's health and effectively treat liver disease.

Tips and Tricks from Those Who've Made a Successful Change

Making a successful lifestyle change, particularly in terms of nutrition and health, is a journey that many people start but do not finish. Those that do frequently share common tactics and mindsets that aid in overcoming the hurdles connected with such substantial transformations. Here are practical advice and insightful methods gathered from people who have successfully modified their diets and lives, especially to help novices on their own paths to health and wellbeing.

1. Start Small.

Many great tales begin with incremental, attainable modifications rather than major overhauls. For example, adding a salad to your daily meals or replacing soda with water might gradually lead to more significant improvements. These little stages are less scary and more sustainable in the long run.

2. Plan Your Meals.

Meal planning is an important practice that many successful people credit with helping them get where they are today. Planning your meals allows you to avoid the traps of last-minute decisions and quick food. Take some time each weekend to plan out your meals for the week ahead. Prepare some meals ahead of time, or at least have a clear plan and the necessary items.

3. Keep A Food Diary.

Writing down what you eat every day might help you spot trends and suggest areas for improvement. A meal diary is more than simply counting calories; it's about knowing your routines. You may notice, for example, that you nibble when anxious or skip breakfast when pressed. Recognizing these patterns is the first step toward altering them.

4. Find Supportive Communities.

Many people owe their success to the help of others. This may come from family and friends, as well as online networks and local groups who follow similar routes. Sharing your goals, problems, and triumphs with like-minded others may be extremely motivating and give vital advice and support.

5. Educate Yourself.

Knowledge is power. Understanding the nutritional value of food, the advantages of various diets, and the effects of specific foods on your health may help you make more educated decisions. Make time to study books, watch documentaries, and follow renowned health and wellness gurus online.

6. Make It Enjoyable.

If you love the procedure, you will be more inclined to remain with it. Find dishes that are not only healthful, but also tasty and enjoyable to prepare. If exercise is part of your lifestyle shift, find activities that you truly like. If you despise your exercises or meals, you're less likely to stick to your schedule.

7. Set Realistic Goals.

Goal setting may help you keep focused and motivated, but it's critical that your goals are attainable. Unrealistic objectives can cause disillusionment and disrupt your development. Set goals that will push you without setting you up for failure. Celebrate tiny triumphs along the road to keep your spirits up.

8. Be Flexible.

Life is unpredictable, and flexibility is essential for sticking to your lifestyle adjustments despite life's ups and downs. If you miss a workout or eat too much at a party, don't consider it a failure. Acknowledge your mistake, learn from it if feasible, and then get back on track.

9. Learn to Handle Setbacks.

Setbacks are a regular part of life, and they are especially common when undertaking major changes. Instead of being hard on yourself or giving up, view failures as learning opportunities. Analyze what caused the setback and how you might avoid such circumstances in the future.

10. Prioritize Your Well-Being.

Above all, successful people put their health and well-being first. This includes not just concentrating on nutrition and exercise, but also getting enough sleep, controlling stress, and obtaining expert medical assistance as needed.

CONCLUSION

As we finish the pages of this cookbook, I'd want to express my deepest gratitude to you, our readers. By bringing this book into your homes and lives, you have not only invested in your health and well-being, but you have also joined a community devoted to adopting a healthier lifestyle via mindful eating and living. Your decision to participate in our work demonstrates not just a passion for tasty, nutritious food, but also a dedication to live a life full of vibrant health and wellbeing.

This cookbook was produced for two purposes. First, to provide delicious recipes that promote liver health and general well-being, and second, to serve as a guide for changing eating habits in ways that feed both the body and spirit. Every dish, piece of advice, and nutritional insight has been meticulously chosen to provide you with the skills you need to make informed, health-promoting decisions on a daily basis.

Your journey through these pages is about more than just following recipes; it's about creating a lifestyle that values nutritious and tasty meals as the foundation of good health. We've journeyed together through chapters that have hopefully informed, taught, and inspired, from grasping the complicated links between nutrition and liver health to discovering how simple, enjoyable activities like cooking may have a significant influence on your well-being.

The Gift of Feedback

In exchange for incorporating these meals and recommendations into your routine, we kindly want feedback. If you've found this cookbook useful, please consider providing an honest star rating and review on the site where you purchased it. Your input is not only critical for helping others discover and use this material; it is also vital to us as writers.

Reviews and ratings do more than only raise our book's visibility; they also give us with valuable information regarding your experiences. Each evaluation helps us learn what works, what resonates, and where we can improve. This input is important since it informs future initiatives and allows us to adjust our writing to your expectations and needs. Your candid feedback and compliments help us improve our future work and make it more aligned with what you, as a reader and home cook, want to see on your shelves.

A Plea for Community Support

In the world of writing and publishing, exposure is essential. Every review you give helps our book stand out in a crowded market. By sharing your views and evaluations, you help others like yourself discover and benefit from our recipes and advice. This act of sharing your views broadens the scope of our community and builds a larger, more connected group of health-conscious individuals.

Furthermore, your input acts as a lighthouse for us, leading the creation of fresh material that meets your requirements and interests. Whether you're suggesting new subjects, nutritional themes, or types of recipes, your feedback helps us understand what you need and how we can meet it.

Looking forward

As we look ahead, we are committed to continue our path of health education and gastronomic enjoyment. Every day, we are motivated by reader tales about how they have improved their cooking habits and, as a result, their health. Your triumphs inspire us to innovate, explore farther, and strive for greatness in every dish and word we create.

We are ready to adapt, enhance, and expand our products to guarantee that each iteration of our work meets the highest culinary and nutritional standards. Your participation in this journey through feedback and interaction is not just desired; it is required.

Thank you.

Thank you again, from the bottom of our hearts, for purchasing this cookbook. We hope it benefits you by bringing health, pleasure, and wonderful meals to your table. Remember, each step you take in following these recipes is a step toward a healthy life, and each review you give illuminates the path for all of us.

Let us continue to cook, eat, and thrive.

With heartfelt thanks and happy wishes,

Anita Jacobs.

www.ingramcontent.com/pod-product-compliance
Lightning Source LLC
Chambersburg PA
CBHW081649260726
48653CB00009BA/3322